CRISTOFANO
AND THE PLAGUE

A study in the history of Public Health
in the age of Galileo

CRISTOFANO AND THE PLAGUE

*A study in the history of Public Health
in the age of Galileo*

CARLO M. CIPOLLA

COLLINS
ST JAMES'S PLACE, LONDON
1973

William Collins Sons & Co Ltd
London · Glasgow · Sydney · Auckland
Toronto · Johannesburg

First published 1973
© Carlo M. Cipolla 1973

ISBN 0 00 211191 8

Set in Monotype Bembo
Made and printed in Great Britain by
William Collins Sons & Co Ltd Glasgow

CONTENTS

ILLUSTRATIONS

PREFACE

There are numerous histories of plague and of individual epidemics – local or widespread. However, this is not – nor does it set out to be – a history of a plague in the traditional sense. At least in the intention of its author, what follows is rather the story of a small band, caught in a tragic crisis – and of the way in which they reacted to it. They were men – with their virtues and their defects. There were no saints. Some however responded much better than others. The tragedy gave the opportunity to some to show initiative, courage, civic sense, humanity. But at the same time tragedy and death were not enough to eliminate from the hearts of people pettiness and avarice. In the background operated a highly developed organization of Public Health, whose action however was frustrated by the medical ignorance and the economic poverty of a pre-industrial society.

ACKNOWLEDGEMENTS

This is the list of people whom I plagued incessantly in the course of my research. First of all I must mention Prof. G. Pampaloni, Director of the Archivio di Stato of Florence, Prof. F. Melis, Dr M. Spallanzani, Miss E. Cecchi, Mr A. Brizzi of the Archivio di Stato of Prato and last but not least my friend M. Bernocchi. I also received precious help from the Azienda Autonoma Provinciale del Turismo in Prato and I wish to express my gratitude to Mr O. Magistrali, Prof. M. Santi, Mr M. Bellandi and Mr C. Paoletti. I pestered Professors M. Abrate and G. Levi in Turin, Professors G. L. Basini and M. Romani in Parma, Prof. E. Fiumi in Volterra, Professors G. Cozzi and F. Seneca in Padua, Prof. Möller in Pavia and I reached also the obliging directors of the Public Libraries of Ancona, Belluno, Ferrara, La Spezia, Livorno, Perugia, Pisa, Ravenna, Sondrio, Trento and Udine. Pitiless as *Pasteurella pestis* I did not spare the loving members of my family, in particular my wife Ora and my brother Manlio. My wife had literally to live with a subject which is not congenial to her gentle nature and yet she gave me all sorts of useful advice about style and composition. A humanist, a medical doctor and a learned bacteriologist my brother provided me with invaluable help for the understanding of disease and the behaviour of epidemics in general.

My secretary Franca Zennaro is perhaps the chief victim. Although she had been immunized by previous action, I doubt that she will ever recover again from this experience.

Dr G. Hutchings revised the entire text and translated large portions from the Italian into English. My good and tolerant friend Richard Ollard took excellent care of this book from its earliest and rough draft until its final form.

ACKNOWLEDGEMENTS

All these people have suffered enough. There is no reason to add to their afflictions by making them responsible for the errors that the book may contain.

The research was made possible by a grant from the Italian National Council for Research (Consiglio Nazionale delle Ricerche) which with contract No. 70.02244.10 put at my disposal all necessary funds.

ABBREVIATIONS

Used in the footnotes for reference to documentation

ACM = Archivio Storico Civico di Milano.

ACP = Archivio Comunale di Pavia.

ACT = Archivio Comunale di Torino.

ASF = Archivio di Stato di Firenze.

ASM = Archivio di Stato di Milano.

ASP = Archivio di Stato di Prato.

ASP, *Diurno* 2=Archivio di Stato di Prato, *Fondo Comunale*, b. 225. Diurno 2 del Cancelliere V. Mainardi.

ASP, *Diurno* 3=Archivio di Stato di Prato, *Fondo Comunale*, b. 226. Diurno 3 del Cancelliere V. Mainardi.

ASP, LS=Archivio di Stato di Prato, *Fondo Comunale*, b. 4047. Libro della Sanità di Cristofano di Giulio Ceffini.

NOTE

All the Tuscan documents referred to in this book carry dates in the Florentine calendar (*calculus florentinus*) of the Incarnation (*annus incarnationis dominicae*).

As against the modern calendar, the Florentine year began on 25th March, i.e. two months, twenty-five days later than our year. Thus the actual Florentine year coincided with our modern notation from 25th March to 31st December, while from 1st January to 24th March it is one year short of ours. A Florentine document dated 2nd Feb. 1629 will therefore correspond to 2nd Feb. 1630 by our calendar.

In the following pages, all dates have been changed from Florentine to modern notation.

CHAPTER I

THE BACKGROUND

Between 1613 and 1666, Europe was devastated by a dreadful series of plague epidemics. According to George Sticker, the epidemics of 1613-35 were part of a cycle that he labelled 'Indian' because of its possible distant origin in India in 1611; the epidemics of 1636-66 he distinguished as 'Levantine' because they allegedly originated in Constantinople in 1636.[1] Classifications are often useful but more often they are arbitrary. It is not altogether impossible that all the epidemics of plague which occurred during the entire period 1613-66 belonged to one single pandemic cycle which swept across the European subcontinent through an intricate network of channels of infection. Whatever the origin, the diffusion and severity of the plague were certainly intensified by the state of endemic war that prevailed in Europe between 1618 and 1659.[2] As usual the folly of man contributed to the deadly action of the microbes.

In September 1629 a German army moved into Italy marching toward Mantua. The troops entered Italy via the St Gothard pass and moved south along Lake Como. 'Most of these Germans are infected with plague because of their wantonness and their dirtiness' wrote Dr Tadino, a physician and Public Health officer of the time.[3] From the houses and the villages in which the German soldiers quartered came

1. STICKER, *Pest*, pp. 128-74.
2. PRINZING, *Epidemics*, chapt. 3, pp. 25-78.
3. TADINO, *Raguaglio*, p. 13.

'unbearable odours due to the rotting straw whereon they sleep and die'.[1]

At that time Italy was probably the best organized country in Europe in regard to the control of Public Health. That keen English traveller and observer, Fynes Moryson, who knew at first hand most of Europe and the Near East, wrote at the beginning of the seventeenth century: 'They (the Italians) are carefull to avoyde infection of the plague and to that purpose in every citty have Magistrates for Health.'[2] But a crude and tough soldiery bent on 'robbing and burning houses and many other excesses' was not likely to abide by the wide orders and controls of the Health officers. 'The German soldiers roam without health passes and they stay wheresoever they will,' remarked Dr Tadino with a note of bitterness and a touch of naiveté.[3] Italians rarely agree on anything, but in this instance, once the plague had been recognized as such, almost everybody agreed that it had been brought into Italy by the German soldiery. We have no reason to question this view,[4] but we cannot be sure it was the whole truth. In 1628 and 1629 the plague ravaged Lyon and a number of places in Provence, Languedoc and Savoy.[5] By October 1629 it was recognized on the Italian side of the Alpine region in Brianzone, San Michele della Chiusa and Chiomonte. When on November 23rd a young man fell suddenly ill in Turin, the rumour spread that

1. TADINO, *Raguaglio*, p. 26.

2. MORYSON, *Itinerary* (ed. 1903), p. 460.

3. TADINO, *Raguaglio*, p. 26 and also p. 77.

4. According to PRINZING, *Epidemics*, p. 40 'during this time, from 1625 to 1630 when epidemics were raging almost everywhere in North Germany, South Germany also suffered, since diseases were often brought there by Imperialist troops and wandering rabble. A pestilence in Augsburg (1628) became very widespread'.

5. GRILLOT, *Lyon;* RAVASINI, *Documenti sanitari,* p. 14; DE SAINT GENIS, *Savoie,* p. 291.

it was the plague. The young man recovered,[1] but the Health
Board of Milan did not want to take chances: on December
5th, it quarantined not only Savoy and other parts of Piedmont
but also the town of Turin.[2] The measure was drastic but not
absurd. In the second part of January 1630, another suspicious
case occurred in Turin[3] and by early spring the plague reached
epidemic proportions in Turin as well as in many other parts of
Piedmont.[4] All evidence seems to indicate that the plague
crossed the Alps from the West with the French soldiery as it
did from the North with the German troops.

Misfortunes never come single. A series of unfortunate circumstances contributed to the appalling diffusion of the
disease. In 1628 and 1629 Northern Italy had been stricken by
an extremely severe famine. Plague depends more on the supply
of rats and fleas than on people's hunger, but there is no doubt
that an impoverished and undernourished population offers
less resistance to the onslaught of the disease. Other factors may
have been involved. Dr Fiochetto mentions 'the humidity and
the great rains of 1629'.[5] He supposed a direct influence of the
weather on human bodies; we may suppose that humidity
possibly favoured the growth of the flea population, although
this, too, is debatable. A more interesting piece of information
is supplied by an anonymous writer who described the course
of the plague in the little town of Busto Arsizio, between Como
and Milano. He noticed that 'in 1630 . . . there prevailed such a
great quantity of rats that people could hardly protect themselves either at daytime or at night from the molesting rage of
these animals. Neither was it possible to save anything from

1. CLARETTA, *Municipio Torinese*, p. 25.
2. ASF, *Sanità*, Bandi, t.I, c. 424.
3. FIOCHETTO, *Trattato*, p. 19.
4. FIOCHETTO, *Trattato*; CLARETTA, *Municipio Torinese*; MONTU, *Peste*.
5. FIOCHETTO, *Trattato*, p. 29.

their fury because of their great number. One could count them by the hundreds in every house and they were so big that people went in terror of them. They damaged everything and especially woollens and linens and they were so hungry that they gnawed at doors and windows . . .'[1] The author did not suspect any link between the expansion of the murine population and the spread of plague and we do not know whether the phenomenon that he described was limited to Busto Arsizio or had a more general character.

The territories of Lake Como were part of the State of Milan.

The news of the outbreak of the plague in the north-eastern territories of Lake Como reached Milan on the 21st of October 1629.[2] October 21st was a Sunday[3] and the officers of the Public Health Board were in their villas in the country. Recalled to Milan they probably met on the 22nd.[4] On October 24th a Florentine observer reported that so far the Health Board had not yet taken any precautions.[5] Criticism is always easier than action. Drastic measures in the field of public health had far reaching consequences on all aspects of human activity and especially on the economy. Before taking such measures the Board wanted to be fully informed. First it rushed Commissioner Cisero to the spot with a physician, then, one or two days later, it delegated physician Tadino to inspect the area in the company of a jurist in order not only to ascertain the facts but also to take such local measures and issue such orders as the situation required.[6] On October 29th the Board received confirmation from Dr Tadino that the plague

1. JOHNSSON, *Busto Arsizio*, p. 63.   2. NICOLINI, *Peste*, pp. 80-81.
3. CAPPELLI, *Cronologia*, p. 85.   4. NICOLINI, *Peste*, p. 81.
5. NICOLINI, *Peste*, p. 82.
6. TADINO, *Raguaglio*, p. 24; NICOLINI, *Peste*, pp. 82-83.

was rampant in the territories of Lake Como.[1] On the same day and the following one, the Board issued drastic orders to prevent the spread of the disease – guards at all the gates of Milan, reinforcement of the laws on the use of health passes in all territories of the State, health controls on all movements of people and merchandise, orders to all Communities with more than 50 families to enclose their inhabitated areas and to barricade the gates, an injunction to physicians, surgeons and barbers to report all deaths of a suspicious nature to the Public Health officers immediately.[2]

In the course of the month of October[3], a soldier coming from Lecco had entered Milan, carrying with him articles of clothing which he had bought or stolen from the German troops. After his arrival in Milan he fell ill and was brought to the hospital. He showed 'a tumour at the elbow of the left arm, a very malignant bubo in the armpit and developed pestilential fever; on the fourth day, death followed'. To avoid the rigours of the Health Board, the family of the soldier contended that the soldier's illness and death had been caused by 'the long journey and the effort of carrying so many things'. The Health officers did not listen to such arguments

1. TADINO, *Raguaglio*, p. 25.

2. For all these points see TADINO, *Raguaglio*, p. 27; NICOLINI, *Peste*, pp. 90-91; *Grida generale per introdurre in tutto lo Stato di Milano l'uso delle bollette personali di Sanità e di metter i rastelli a tutti li luoghi da cinquanta fuochi in su*, 30th Oct. 1629 (a copy also in ACP, b. 445); *Grida per notificare quelli che moriranno subitamente o in tre o quattro giorni o che ne i loro corpi si scoprirà qualche segno dubbioso di infettione*, 30th Oct. 1629 (a copy also in ACP, b. 445).

3. According to TADINO, *Raguaglio*, pp. 50-1 the soldier came to Milan on October 22nd but in ACM, *Materie*, Epidemie, b. 349 is preserved the official report about the death of the soldier. The report is dated October 16th. See also GHIRON, *Documenti*, pp. 753-4.

and all the belongings of the soldier and his bed were burned.[1] But it did not help. Sporadic cases of plague kept cropping up in Milan during the winter, and with the arrival of spring the epidemic erupted in all its violence, reaching its climax during the summer.[2] June, July and August were the worst months. When the epidemic broke out, Milan had about 130,000 inhabitants. By the end of August 1630, more than 60,000 people had died.[3] Apocalyptic as they are, these figures still do not convey completely all the human horrors experienced in those dreadful months by the Lombard metropolis. From the beginning of September 1630, the epidemic subsided in Milan,[4] but in the meantime it had spread through Northern and Central Italy.

Despite being divided into a number of independent states, Italy possessed a very efficient network of information in regard to Public Health. The news of the outbreak of the plague in the northern part of Lake Como first reached Milan on October 21st, 1629. By October 26th most towns in Northern and Central Italy were already in a state of alarm, and soon measures were taken. On October 27th Venice decreed the ban of the territories of Lecco, Risano and Chiuso which meant that neither people nor merchandise were allowed to go to or come from the banished territories. The same measure was taken by Verona on October 29th, by Bologna on October 31st, by Piacenza on November 7th, by Modena and Florence on November 8th, by Ancona on November 11th.[5] In the meantime it became known that the plague had spread

1. TADINO, *Raguaglio*, pp. 50-51 and GHIRON, *Documenti*, pp. 753-4.
2. RIPAMONTI, *De Peste*, p. 68; TADINO, *Raguaglio*, pp. 115, 117.
3. BESTA, *Popolazione di Milano*, p. 9; SELLA, *Popolazione*, pp. 464-5.
4. TADINO, *Raguaglio*, p. 134.
5. ASF, *Sanità*, Bandi, t.I, cc. 414-419. For Piacenza, ACP, b. 444.

to other areas of the State of Milan and that, as a decree issued in Verona reported, 'in the very town of Milan some people died in the main hospital of that city with obvious signs of contagion'. On November 8th, Verona decreed the ban of the whole State of Milan.[1] Modena extended the original ban of Lecco, Risano and Chiuso to a number of other places in the State of Milan on November 19th. Piacenza did likewise on November 23rd and on December 9th, Bologna on December 16th, Florence on December 29th, Rome on January 3rd, 1630.[2] Despite all precautions, however, the plague broke through the defences hurriedly erected by the Health officers of the various places. The maps on p. 22 show the timing and the geography of its devastating progress. Brescia, Mantua, Verona, Vicenza, Padua, Venice, Pavia, Piacenza, Parma, Reggio, Modena, Bologna, Turin, all fell prey to the plague and every place experienced the same horrors and the same terrors.

In the case of plague as in most diseases, treatment was of no value in general and occasionally it was harmful. Gastaldi, the bright and energetic cardinal who was put in charge of the Health Board in Rome during the plague of 1656-7 wrote in his famous *Treatise on Plague* that 'the writings of doctors on the cure of plague produce much smoke and offer little light. Medical remedies against the plague have been proven by practice to be of no use and at times dangerous',[3] As people

1. ASF, *Sanità*, Bandi, t.I, c. 413. The decree is mistakenly dated '8th October 1629, Thursday'. In the same decree reference is made to the previous decree of 'the 29th of last October'. Moreover, Oct. 8th 1629 was a Friday while Nov. 8th was a Thursday (CAPPELLI, *Cronologia*, p. 85).

2. ASF, *Sanità*, Bandi, t.I, cc. 420-440.

3. GASTALDI, *Tractatus*, pp. 2-4.

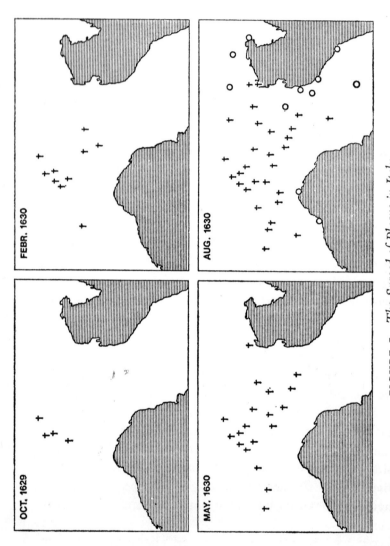

OCT. 1629

FEBR. 1630

MAY. 1630

AUG. 1630

FIGURE 1 . *The Spread of Plague in Italy*

The crosses indicate major towns hit by the plague. Circles indicate major towns that escaped the epidemic.

commonly said, the only good remedy against the plague were 'pills made of three ingredients called, *cito*, *longe* and *tarde* (swiftly, far, and tardily), namely run swiftly, go far and return tardily'.[1]

Diagnosis was undoubtedly more advanced than therapy, but still far from being satisfactory. Physicians and surgeons could recognize bubonic plague, but they had no objective criteria for the diagnosis of the pneumonic and septicaemic forms. In fact, as Dr Ingrassia wrote in the sixteenth century, 'many physicians mistakenly report that plague is not present when they do not see buboes, anthraxes, papules, sports or similar signs on the bodies of the deceased'.[2]

More advanced than both therapy and diagnosis was the body of rules and practices designed to prevent and/or control the spread of the disease. Physicians and Health officers still believed in the influence of the heavenly bodies, and discussing the origin of the plague of 1630 the learned Dr Tadino of Milan wrote that 'at that time Saturn and Jupiter were in conjunction and this fact was a warning that the year 1630 was to produce mortal diseases'.[3] However, even though they emphatically believed in the influence of the conjunctions of the heavenly bodies, Health officers, physicians and surgeons did not actually credit them with any other significance than that of creating a favourable predisposition for the outbreak of the disaster. With equal conviction they admitted that the disease essentially occurred because of, and spread by, contagion; and, as the learned archbishop of Milan wrote, 'contagion can occur by contact or by breath'.[4] The first thing to do therefore, in case of plague, was to keep healthy people away

1. INGRASSIA, *Informatione*, part I, p. 1.

2. INGRASSIA, *Informatione*, part I, p. 24. Cf. also GALASSI, *Imola*, vol. 2, p. 226.

3. TADINO, *Raguaglio*, p. 15.   4. RIPAMONTI, *De Peste*, pp. 174-5.

from infected people as well as from infected animals and infected objects and to stop trade and communications with infected places. For this purpose Health officers normally resorted to the establishment of sanitary cordons, use of health passes, isolation of infected persons and contacts, and various types of quarantine. These measures had no scientific basis but no one can question their wisdom. Essentially they were the product of common sense, haphazard observation, and the vaguely stated but strongly felt conviction that as far as precautions were concerned too much was better than too little.

A major institution in the public health organization of the time was the lazaretto or pest-house. The lazaretto was a building for isolating people thought to have an infectious disease or to be incubating it, and in the period under consideration the disease most feared was generally the plague. A few major Italian cities had established permanent pest-houses at an early date. The two most famous lazarettos of this kind were those of Venice and Milan and both had been built in the course of the fifteenth century. Yet, permanent pest-houses were still a rarity in early seventeenth century Europe. There was no permanent pest-house in London or elsewhere in England in 1630 and several years were to pass before the state officially advocated the provision of permanent pest-houses. In Italy, too, most of the towns, including large and famous ones such as Florence and Bologna had no permanent lazarettos.[1] If an epidemic developed, a large and commodious building, possibly outside the walls of the town, was requisitioned and made into a pest-house.

While in England pest-houses generally lacked medical and

1. For Florence Catellacci, *Ricordi*, pp. 382-4; for Bologna Brighetti, *Bologna*, pp. 77 ff.

nursing attendance,[1] these services were generally provided in the Italian lazarettos. In the pest-houses of small towns normally a surgeon was considered adequate for attending the sick. In larger pest-houses a staff of both physicians and surgeons was considered indispensable. In the lazaretto at San Miniato in Florence, early in November 1630 there were two physicians and nine surgeons in addition to a lay personnel of 134 people and 5 friars[2]; but as the number of patients amounted to almost 800 a raising of the number of both doctors and surgeons was recommended.[3] Among others a female surgeon – Margarita di Giovanni Lombardi – was added to the staff to take care of the female patients.[4]

It was not easy however to find people willing to serve in the pest-houses. Everybody resisted confinement to that inferno and with few notable exceptions the physicians, being people of high social standing and good economic condition, resisted more than the others. Dr Tadino reports extensively about the difficulties of finding physicians for the pest-house in Milan during the plague of 1630.[5] In Florence, in 1630, the College of Physicians hesitated to appoint two of its members to serve in the lazaretto at San Miniato. When the Health Board reiterated its request with tones of urgency, the College tactfully declared its readiness to examine all doctors and surgeons whom the Board would compel to come to Florence from other cities of the Grand Duchy to serve in the pest-house.[6] In Rome during the plague of 1656-7 'high fees and special prizes were not enough to induce doctors to go

1. SHREWSBURY, Bubonic Plague, p. 354.
2. ASF, Sanità, Negozi, b. 152, c. 461 and 478 (10th Nov. 1630).
3. ASF, Sanità Negozi, b. 152, c. 492 (11th Nov. 1630).
4. ASF, Sanità, Negozi, b. 156, c. 855 (23rd April 1631).
5. TADINO, Raguaglio, pp. 105-6.
6. ASF, Sanità, Negozi, b. 151, c. 1087; Copialettere, b. 56, c. 5v-6.

and tend people in the pest-houses and they had to be compelled to do so by public authority.'[1] In Bologna during the plague of 1630 a petition addressed to the Health Office by the local physicians emphasized that 'for doctors to go and serve in the lazarettos is like going to certain death' and it gave evidence of eight physicians who had died in the pest-houses in slightly more than two months. The physicians suggested that the patients ought to be cured at a distance, with the barber-surgeon of the lazaretto shouting out of the windows 'the quality, sex, condition of the patient and the stage of the illness'. From a safe distance the doctor would shout back the cure. Thus 'the patients would receive the proper treatment and physicians would not die'.[2] It might seem a little odd that while the physicians were reluctant to move to the pest-houses, they should take it for granted that the surgeons would accept the frontline post. But physicians and surgeons came from and belonged to quite different social classes and in those days the value attributed to human life largely depended on class and social status.

When an epidemic broke out and the number of patients increased rapidly, a pest-house inevitably suffered from shortages of beds, blankets, mattresses, fire wood, medicine and sometimes food. In San Miniato at Florence, early in November 1630, in the women's section there were 412 female patients and only 82 beds; as the report says 'at present there is an average of five women who must sleep in the same bed'. In the men's section, there were 93 beds and 312 patients.[3]

1. GASTALDI, *Tractatus*, pp. 4-5.
2. BRIGHETTI, *Bologna*, pp. 110-252. The practice suggested by the physicians of Bologna in 1630 had been followed in Milan during the plague of 1576, cf. BELLENTANI, *Dialogo*, p. 297.
3. ASF, *Sanità*, Negozi, b. 152, c. 461 (10th Nov. 1630).

Indeed, in times of epidemics a pest-house offered a preview of hell. When the President of the Milanese Board of Public Health, G. B. Arconato visited the pest-house of Milan during the famine of 1629 'he went into a dead faint for the stinking smells that came forth from all those bodies and those little rooms'.[1] Cardinal Spada reporting on the conditions of the pest-houses of Bologna during the plague of 1630 recorded that 'here you see people lament, others cry, others strip themselves to the skin, others die, others become black and deformed, others lose their minds. Here you are overwhelmed by intolerable smells. Here you cannot walk but among corpses. Here you feel naught but the constant horror of death. This is the faithful replica of hell since here there is no order and only horror prevails'.[2]

Normally besides the lazarettos for the infected there were also pest-houses for the convalescents. These establishments were not set up to help the convalescents in their recovery but to keep them in isolation for a further period after they had been removed from the crowd of the sick. It was generally believed that once recovered a convalescent could still be infectious for some time. This was a sound and perfectly correct idea, but in the absence of microscopy and microbiological knowledge, it remained at the level of ingenious intuition and could not possibly develop into a scientifically tested criterion. The basic rule was that the longer the period of isolation, the greater the margin of safety. This often caused great injustice to the patients but as a Health officer wrote in our own times, until one has satisfactory methods of laboratory examinations, one must 'attempt to sail that difficult course between too great risk to the community and too great an injustice to the

1. TADINO, *Raguaglio*, p. 11.   2. BRIGHETTI, *Bologna*, p. 80

patients. Lucky is the Health officer who can avoid both Scylla and Charybdis'.

A distinction was always drawn between the 'infected' and the 'suspect'. 'Infected' was any sick person whose illness had been diagnosed as plague by a physician or by a surgeon. 'Suspect' was anybody who had been in contact with an infected person or with infected objects (today we would call such a person a 'contact') and also anybody coming from an area which was thought to harbour the plague.

Modern epidemiologists insist that 'on no account should patients and contacts be locked up in an infected house as was done in the Middle Ages and repeated as late as 1921 in Manchuria'.[1] The advantage of removing an infected person from a house does not need to be explained. The advantage of rapidly removing contacts is that incipient cases may be quickly detected before they become infectious. All this was known in seventeenth-century Italy. Not only was it universally recognized that the infected people should be isolated in the pesthouses, but it was also recommended that the contacts be isolated in special quarters separated from the healthy as well as the infected. On May 23rd 1630, the President and Officers of the Health Board of Milan warned that 'if the contacts remain confined in their homes they will be dangerous to themselves and to the others'.[2] In Rome in 1656, Cardinal Gastaldi noted that by forcing also the contacts of high rank into special pest-houses mortality among them was reduced to less than five per cent.[3] In a permanent pest-house such as that of Milan, there were distinct quarters for the infected and for the sus-

1. WU, *Plague*, p. 476.
2. ASM, *Sanità*, Parte antica, b. 286.
3. GASTALDI, *Tractatus*, p. 90.

pects.[1] Where no permanent pest-houses were available, during epidemics the Public Health authorities generally aimed at establishing separate pest-houses for the infected and for the contacts.

Unfortunately social privileges and financial difficulties often stood in the way of the aims and plans of the Health officers. 'People greatly fear being moved to the lazaretto,' wrote Cardinal Gastaldi. To break the resistance of the poor was not so difficult. To break the resistance of the wealthy and powerful was quite another matter. Not all infected people were sent to the pest-house and when lack of funds prevented the establishment of separate pest-houses the contacts were locked in their homes.[2]

When a case of plague occurred and was recognized as such, the house was locked up. If people were segregated inside, the Health authorities had three main preoccupations:

(a) to ensure that people inside would not come in contact with people outside;

(b) to provide the people inside with the supplies necessary for their survival;

1. TADINO, *Raguaglio*, pp. 58–9.

2. On occasion the contacts were confined together with the infected in one pest-house with disastrous results. BELLENTANI, *Dialogo*, p. 298 wrote: 'I saw in the above mentioned cities (Brescia and Marseilles) carts whereon ten or twelve persons were brought to the pest-house and out of them only one was perhaps infected; the others were suspects. Since the two groups were put together hugger-mugger in the pest-house, it followed that in eight to ten days all became infected and died. On the contrary I saw in Milan groups of 50 to 60 being brought to the pest-house and one of them was infected. This one was set apart in the infirmary. The suspects were quarantined in different quarters and, thanks to God, they remained healthy.'

CRISTOFANO AND THE PLAGUE

(c) to provide for the disinfection of the house and of the household items.[1]

To take care of the first problem, the doors of the house were nailed or bolted on the outside. Alternatively guards were posted at the doors. In both cases the doors were also marked for the purpose of scaring away passers-by.[2] It is amazing yet all too true to human nature that even in such horrible circumstances people managed to turn the different ways of confinement into symbols of social discrimination. In Turin, the members of the upper classes 'did not suffer' being bolted in their homes and wanted guards at their doors, a privilege that the city granted on condition that the guarded would pay for their guards.[3]

Supplies were obtained by those inside by lowering a basket from the window to the street below where it was filled with necessities.[4] In the case of wealthy people it was generally

1. This was done also when there were no people segregated in the infected house.

2. Doors were marked with a red cross in Modena in 1630 (SERRA, *Modena*, pp. 108 and 131) and in Padua in 1631 (FERRARI, *Ufficio della Sanità*, p. 125), with a white cross in Verona in 1630 (PONA, *Gran Contagio* pp. 37, 55), with the word '*Sanità*' in Florence (RONDINELLI, *Contagio*, pp. 51-2). In London in 1630 the Privy Council directed the Lord Mayor that every infected house in which the occupants were segregated 'should have guards set at the door and a red cross or *Lord have mercy upon us* set on the door to warn passers-by'. (SHREWSBURY, *Bubonic Plague*, p. 355).

3. ACT, *Ordinati*, vol. 149, c. 19, June 20th, 1599. During the plague of 1599 the city council passed an ordnance to the effect that people could not be freed unless they had fully paid the cost of the guards to the city's treasurer. (ACT, *Ordinati*, vol. 149, c. 16, June 19th, 1599). In 1630, Dr Fiochetto complained that there were people who asked for guards and then 'after four or five days they pretend that they are poor and cannot afford to pay' thus trying to have the guards at the expense of the town (FIOCHETTO, *Trattato*, p. 42).

4. When a death occurred in such a house, the body of the deceased was

expected that they should pay for their own supplies. The real problem lay with the provisioning of the common people. One did not have to be 'poor' even by the standards of those days, to find oneself in need of public charity once one's house had been locked up. Craftsmen, labourers, and petty traders had little or no savings: they lived from day to day on what they earned,[1] and once in confinement they had to be supported at the expense of the community.[2]

As to disinfection of buildings, it was done in general by washing the walls and floor with vinegar, by application of lime and by the burning of sulphur. The wealthy would also use odoriferous substances which were as costly as they were useless. Once disinfected and perfumed, the room or rooms so treated had to be sealed off from the rest of the house. The disinfection of the dwellings of the poor was carried out at the city's expense. The clothing of the deceased, as well as his bed with the mattress and the linens, were normally and immediately burned, also at the city's expense.

It is implicit in all that has been said so far that from the onset of an epidemic the problem that the authorities had to face was not only medical and hygienic but also economic. Public funds had to be provided for the setting up and maintaining of the pest-houses, for hiring public doctors, surgeons, grave-

---

also lowered through the window to the street. Such a macabre scene can be observed in a painting preserved in the Archivio di Stato of Bologna and reproduced in BRIGHETTI, *Bologna*, p. 217.

1. '*S'andavan mantenendo alla giornata*' a document of 1630 says of the working population: ACT, *Ordinati*, vol. 179, c. 36, July 20th, 1630.

2. Sometimes the provisions were delivered free to the poor and on a loan basis to those who were considered able to refund the city for the supplies.

diggers, cleaners, guards and the like, for the disinfections and fumigations, for supporting those who were segregated in their homes and could not pay for their maintenance, for reimbursing the poor for the burning of their infected commodities, and for numerous other needs.

As the epidemic developed the economic problems became more and more severe. The cessation of all trade with the outside world deprived the administration of the income from indirect taxation. Employment and private incomes were negatively affected and any increase in direct taxation was out of the question. In fact the yield of direct taxes diminished as so many people died and others were impoverished. Thus, as progressively greater burdens were put on the public bodies, fewer funds were available to them through ordinary channels. The administrators were therefore forced to resort to extraordinary measures, such as contracting loans with banks or individuals and/or obtaining subsidies from the central administration or from the Prince. In so far as the local administrators were unsuccessful in raising the necessary funds, they had to limit their action in the field of public health: this meant painful decisions about alternative measures all of which were or were thought to be tragically indispensable.

CHAPTER II

A COMMUNITY AGAINST
THE PLAGUE

In the spring of 1594 a cultivated English traveller visiting
Tuscany planned his journey from Florence to Pisa. The
distance between the two towns is about 55 miles but he
decided to make 'this journey on foot, meaning leisurely to
see the next Cities, so little distant one from the other, as they
were pleasant journeys on foot, especially in so pleasant a
country'.

The first town he encountered in the first day of his journey
was the 'Castle Prato'. Prato is a Tuscan town, about 13 miles
north-west of Florence. As Fynes Moryson saw it, 'this pleasant
Castle (or walled town) is of a round forme, having at the very
entrance, a large market place, wherein stands a faire Cathed-
rall Church, adorned with many stones of marble'.[1] Another
English traveller who visited Tuscany in 1596, Robert Dallington, recorded:

There are in Italy among I know not how many thousands, foure
principall Castles as above the rest reputed, as Leander Alberti in
his view of Italy discourseth: Barletta in Puglia in the Kingdome of
Naples, Fabriana in Marca Anconitana under the State of the
Church, Crema in Lombardia under the Venetians and Prato in
Tuscana under the Great Duke. It is heere to be observed that these
are called Castles not that they be onely fortresses and places of
strength, but that they be large townes fortified with wall and

1. MORYSON, *Itinerary* (ed. 1907), pp. 308-9.

C.P.   33   C

bulwarke and have their territories; they onely want Bishops Seas, wherein they differ from Citties.[1]

Prato lies in a plain bordered on the west by the pleasant hills of Montalbano and on the north and the east by the 'most stony and barren mountaines, which are called Apennine and divide the length of Italy'.[2] In that 'most pleasant plain' vines and mulberry trees, cypresses and rosemary grew in the harmony of nature.[3] As Moryson wrote:

It was called the Valley of Arno, tilled after the manner of Lombardy, bearing Corne and Wine in the same field, all the furrowes being planted with Elmes upon which the Vines grow.[4]

To English eyes the valley looked more like a garden than arable land:

Their valleys indeed are like Gardens, whether you respect the small quantitie of each mans severall, or their diligence in their keeping, or to say truth, the variety of fruits thereof. Going up with another English Gentleman to the top of a steepe hill, some two miles high right over Prato, to give our eye the view of that pleasant valley, we could not discerne any one peece of ground above one acre and a halfe in our opinions (except the Great Dukes pastures about his Pallace of Poggio), all which ground being bare and the hedges

1. DALLINGTON, *Survey of Tuscany*, pp. 15-16. The reference is to L. Alberti, *Descrittione di tutta Italia*. In this book (p. 35 of the Venetian edition of 1551) Alberti writes in fact that '*egli è annoverato Prato fra le quattro Castella volgate d'Italia per la sua grandezza e bellezza. Così si dice Barletta in Puglia, Fabriano nella Marcha, Crema in Lombardia et Prato in Toscana*'.

2. MORYSON, *Itinerary* (ed. 1907), p. 219.

3. Around Prato the cultivation of mulberries and silkworms was very important in the seventeenth century. There must also have been olive trees but most of the oil consumed in Prato came from the territory of Pescia (ASF, *Sanità*, Negozi, b. 152, c. 490).

4. MORYSON, *Itinerary* (ed. 1907), p. 309.

greene with the vines, gave a very pleasant and delightfull prospect, resembling very fitly a Checker Table.[1]

Politically and administratively, Prato was part of the Grand Duchy of Tuscany whose capital was Florence. The town was administered by a Town Council led by the *Priori* and the *Gonfaloniere*. The central authority of the Grand Duke was locally represented by the *Podestà*. The local administration was closely controlled by the central government; however by the early seventeenth century the local administrators were ready to oblige and most willing to prove their deference and obedience to the *Signori* of Florence.

In the first decades of the seventeenth century Prato numbered about 6,000 souls within the walls and about 11,000 souls within its jurisdiction outside the gates.[2] Today Prato boasts a thriving textile industry that exports its products to the four corners of the world. In the fifteenth century Prato was the base of a huge and thriving mercantile firm, the product of the enterprising and managerial genius of Francesco di Marco Datini, 'the Merchant of Prato'. At the beginning of the seventeenth century the great enterprise of Francesco had long since disappeared and the modern textile industry had not yet started. Robert Dallington visiting Prato in 1596 had a general impression of poverty:[3]

1. DALLINGTON, *Survey of Tuscany*, p. 30.

2. FIUMI, *Prato*, pp. 177-80 and NUTI, *Prato*. These modern authors do not seem to have been aware of the report by Dallington, but their conclusions confirm Dallington's statement (*Survey of Tuscany*, p. 15): 'The Contado (the Territory) of this towne is in length eight miles, in bredth foure, in circuite foure and twentie, within which compasse (with those within the Towne) are fiftie nine Churches, eight and thirtie Monasteries and other religious houses and of all sorts of people sixteene thousand, whereof two thousand are religious.'

3. DALLINGTON, *Survey of Tuscany*, pp. 15-16.

Here in Prato is (they say) the Girdle of our Lady brought thither by a merchant from the Indies . . . a Relicke which is shewed to the people with great reverence once in a yeare, that is, on our Ladies day in September in the time of their Faire, and when is most concourse of strangers. There came that day in devotion (to see me, not the Girdle) two English gentlemen my friends; we observed (if it be not impertinent here to remember) that there were in view upon the Market place of people at the shewing of this Relicke about eighteene or twenty thousand, whereof we iudged one halfe to have hattes of strawe and one fourth part to be bare legged; that we know all is not gold in Italy, though many Travellers gazing onely on the beautie of their Citties and the painted surface of their houses, thinke it the onely Paradize of Europe . . . But no marvaile though Prato be poore being so uniustly and cruelly sacked in the yeare 1512 by the Spaniards.

A few figures that I collected and shall comment upon in the second part of Appendix I confirm Dallington's impression.[1] The mass of the people had exceedingly low standards of living, and the peasants who must have flocked around 'the Relicke' when this was shown 'on our Ladies day' were definitely the most destitute part of the population. There were wealthy people of course, but in Tuscany even the wealthy were noted for 'their egregious and incredible parsimony in feeding as also their frugality from extraordinary spending'.[2]

Within parsimonious Tuscany the Pratesi distinguished

1. The remarks by Dallington outraged the Florentine circles. The Tuscan court accused the English author of libel and pressured the English Crown to inquire on the case (on the episode see Crinó, *Documenti*). As far as I can judge, Dallington was a very perceptive observer and the data he quotes are confirmed by other evidence.

2. DALLINGTON, *Survey of Tuscany*, p. 34.

themselves for 'egregious and incredible parsimony' as well as for 'their frugality'.

The first official warning of the danger of plague reached Prato toward the end of October 1629: a letter dated the 26th from the Health officers in Florence instructed the local administration to place guards for health controls. Only five days had passed since the news of the outbreak of plague on the northern side of Lake Como had reached Milan and the action of the Health Board in Florence could not have been more prompt.[1]

In the absence of any knowledge about vaccination, the establishment of a sanitary cordon was the only preventive measure people could resort to besides prayers and processions. In response to the letter from Florence, the town Council of Prato, on October 27th promptly appointed four citizens to the position of 'Officiali di Sanità' (Health officers).

All affairs pertaining to Public Health were placed in their hands and thus the positioning of the guards also.[2] It was customary at the time to have two lines of defence: one at the borders of the territory, at mountain passes and at fords, and the other at the gates of the city. On November 1st, the Officers of Prato wrote to the Officers in Florence that they had complied with the general instructions received on October 26th.[3] On December 27th, in consideration of the very

1. On October 21st the Florentine observer in Milan wrote to Florence reporting that 'this morning the captain of Lecco arrived in great haste to inform His Excellency that yesterday in a village of Valsassina, near Lecco, virulent plague had been ascertained' (NICOLINI, Peste, pp. 80-1).

2. For all the preceding points see ASP, Diurno 2, cc. 67v-68 (27th Oct. 1629).

3. ASP, Diurno 2, cc. 71v-72. They decided to put four guards at the Antella pass, in the mountains of Prato, toward Bologna, and they placed

cold weather, the officers ordered the construction of barracks
for the guards at three of the five gates and also made provision
of one *staio*[1] of embers per day for the guards at each of the
five gates.[2] It was a small ration of fuel, but in those days
people were accustomed to a harsh life. And so the winter
passed.

In May 1630 the news from the north suddenly became very
alarming: the plague had been identified in Bologna.[3] The
immediate reaction of the Health Board in Florence was to
request that all people moving from one place to another
should carry health passes. No one without such a certificate
could be admitted into the territory of the State or into any
walled place. On May 14th the Board instructed the Health
officers in Prato to appoint a person who would issue the passes
for the local people. Within two days the instructions were
carried out.[4]

In the meantime in Bologna the situation had deteriorated
tragically, and on June 12th Florence rushed troops to the

---

guards at the five gates of the city. Later on, at the suggestion of Cristofano
Ceffini, substitute *Provveditore di Palazzo* (the subject of this book: see below
p. 62), the officers changed their plans and placed the border guards at the
Cerbaia instead of the Antella pass (ASP, *Diurno* 2, c. 73v., 6th Nov. 1629).
For the location of these passes see map, between pages 40 and 41.

1. On the *staio* see below Appendix 2. The *staio* was approximately two
thirds of a bushel.

2. ASP, *Diurno* 2, c. 85.

3. BRIGHETTI, *Bologna*, p. 38. Bologna is situated 65 miles north of
Florence.

4. The officers appointed ser Fausto Novellucci to the office (ASP,
Diurno 2, c. 116, 16th May 1630). Ser Fausto was vice-chancellor of the city
(ASP, *Fondo Comunale*, b. 1038, Entrata e Uscita del Camerlengo Generale
1630-1, c. 80). According to the instructions of the Board in Florence the
health passes had to be issued at no cost to the persons who requested them.
As to the salary of ser Fausto, see below, Appendix 1.

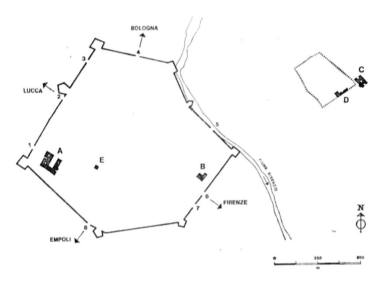

FIGURE 2. *Plan of Prato in the 17th century*

A the hospital *della Misericordia*.
B the hospital of San Sylvester.
C the Convent of St Anne.
D the '*casa del poder murato*'.
E the house of the Ven. Compagnia del Pellegrino.
Gates: 1. San Paolo; 2. Pistoiese; 3. San Fabiano; 4. del Serraglio; 5. Mercatale; 6. Fiorentina; 7. del Soccorso; 8. Santa Trinità.

northern border of the Grand Duchy so that there would be one guard-post every three miles.[1] On the following day, Bologna was put under a total ban, which meant that persons, merchandise and letters could not be received from that city even if accompanied by reassuring health passes.[2] On the 16th all people living close to the border were requested to be on the alert: if they saw strangers crossing the border where there were no guards they had 'to cry in chorus, ring the bells alarmingly

1. ASF, *Sanità*, Copialettere, b. 55, c. 1.
2. ASF, *Sanità*, Copialettere, b. 55, c. 1.

and follow the trespassers until they were captured'.[1] As fear mounted, the activity of Health officers both central and local became feverish. June 16th: the officers of Prato added more guards at the gates and increased the wages of the guards as an obvious incentive to them to be more conscientious;[2] June 22nd: the officers in Florence instructed the Health officers of all towns and walled villages of the Grand Duchy to use greater care in the issuing of health passes;[3] July 1st: the Grand Duke rushed thirty horsemen of his personal guard to strengthen border control;[4] July 6th: the officers in Florence instructed local officers to stop all movements of friars of any religious order;[5] July 10th: in Prato the three most frequently used gates – Mercatale, Fiorentina and Pistoiese – were reinforced with barricades.[6] All in vain.

The establishment of a sanitary cordon is a necessary but rarely sufficient measure. This was especially so in an age when the microbic enemy was unknown and invisible, when animal vectors were not recognized as such and when the reliability and competence of the guards were questionable.

The precautionary measures of the Health officers did not stop the advance of the enemy. By July, the plague had invaded Trespiano, a village four miles north of Florence on the road to Bologna,[7] and by August it had entered the city of

1. ASF, *Sanità*, Copialettere, b. 55, cc. 3-3v.
2. ASP, *Diurno* 2, c. 124.
3. ASF, *Sanità*, Copialettere, b. 55, c. 9.
4. ASF, *Sanità*, Copialettere, b. 55, c. 16v.
5. ASF, *Sanità*, Copialettere, b. 55, c. 21v. Friars served in the pesthouses and they moved around incessantly. On June 21st 1630 also the Health Board of Padua ordered all friars to remain in their convents (FERRARI, *Ufficio della Sanità*, p. 91).
6. ASP, *Diurno* 2, c. 127v.
7. ASF, *Sanità*, Copialettere, b. 55, cc. 62vff. (3rd Aug. 1630), 77v ff. (10th Aug. 1630).

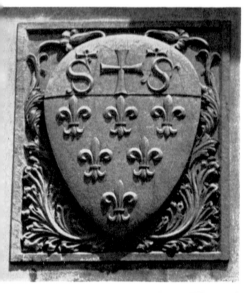

The crest of the hospital of
San Silvestro

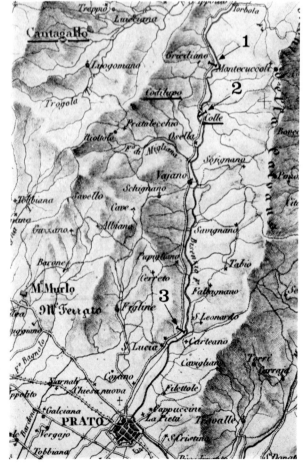

The guard posts at
the approaches to Prato
1 Posto di Cerbaia
2 Ponte a Colle
3 Ponte di Zane
Guards were also posted in
Cantagallo and Codilupo

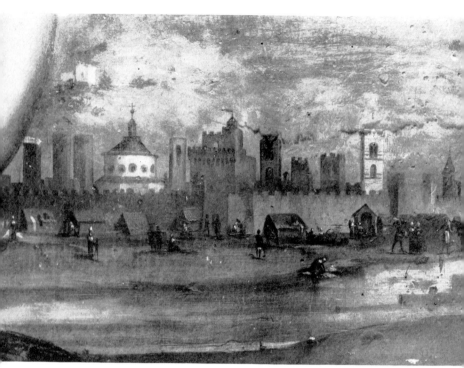

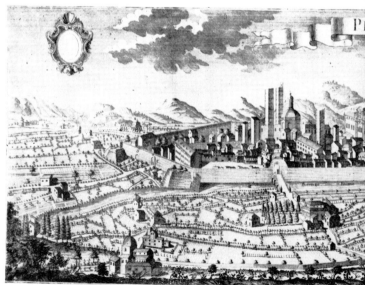

A view of Prato at the beginning of the eighteenth century.
The Convent of St Anne is shown in the lower left foreground

A view of Prato in the early part
of the sixteenth century

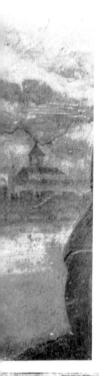

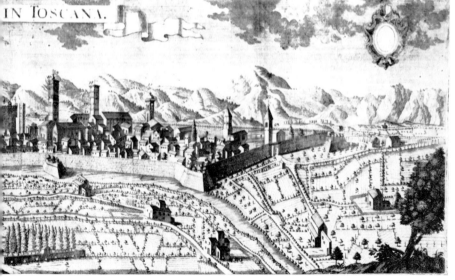

INSTRVZIONE
DEL MAGISTRATO
della Sanità di Firenze.

Per li Rettori di Giustizia di fuori

Ne casi di mali di Contagio, che si sco-prissero nelle loro Iurisdizioni, in particolare per i Contadi, e Ville.

In Firenze, Nella Stamperia di Zanobi Pignoni 1630.

The title page of the instructions issued by the Florentine health authorities

---

Forma di fare le bollette per le persone originarie d'un loco. | *Per le persone che hanno dimorato giorni vinti, o in un loco.* | *Per le persone, che portano le bollette d'altro loco.*

Luoghi sospetti per causa di peste nello Stato di Milano.

Chiuso.	
Malgrate Pieve di Galbiate.	
Castello sopra Adda.	
Bellano.	
Mensio.	
Dorio.	del Cornasco.

Arconatus Praeses.

Città, Provincie, Luoghi sospetti di peste, fuori dello Stato di Milano.

Iacobus Antonius Taliabos Cancell.

The lower part of a decree issued by the Health Board of Milan on 30 October 1629 after plague had been officially recognised in the territories of Lake Como listing the places put under the ban

Florence[1] and Tavola, a little village in the jurisdiction of Prato.[2] Both Trespiano and Tavola were isolated, and in Florence a number of houses were quarantined.[3]

There was resistance to the facts. Physicians kept debating whether it was plague or not, and the Health officers in Florence, pending a final decision, distributed reassuring bulletins deluding themselves and others.[4] But day by day the awful truth became more tragically obvious.

During the months of July and August 1630, mortality in Prato seems to have been higher than normal,[5] and in September there were a number of cases of death and illness of a suspicious nature.[6] The local physicians and surgeons were uncertain in their diagnosis: official confirmation of the plague was resisted because of its disastrous implications, yet the local administration grew increasingly nervous. On August 3rd, 1630, the town council decided to raise the number of the Health officers from four to eight,[7] and about one month later the officers wrote to the Health Board in Florence asking for authorization to prepare a pest-house as a precautionary measure. This was an excellent idea but unfortunately the officers in Florence, in their eagerness to prevent panic and avoid the banning of Tuscany by other states, discouraged the

1. ASF, *Sanità*, Copialettere, b. 55, cc. 101v ff. (31st Aug. 1630).

2. ASF, *Sanità*, Copialettere, b. 55, c. 101 (31st Aug. 1630).

3. ASF, *Sanità*, Copialettere, b. 55, cc. 107v-109 (3rd Sept. 1630). According to this letter 28 houses were quarantined in Florence.

4. ASF, *Sanità*, Copialettere, c. 102v-103 (31st August 1630), c. 107v-109 (3rd Sept.), c. 117v. (7th Sept.), c. 132v-133 (14th Sep .), etc.

5. See below, pp. 70-1 and p. 96 n. 1.

6. ASF, *Sanità*, Negozi, b. 150, c. 971 (19th Sept. 1630).

7. ASP, *Diurno* 2, c. 133v.

initiative. They pointed out that Florence was very close and could easily provide advice and assistance; moreover, the recent rains – they added – by refreshing the air, were bound to have beneficial effects.[1]

Their optimism was ill founded. One man, Niccolò Bardazzi, attendant in the hospital of the Misericordia in Prato was in charge of those cases of death or sickness which looked suspicious. On September 16th the man fell sick and he died on the 19th. This time the physicians had no doubts: it was the plague. The same day the officers of Prato hurriedly reported the facts to those in Florence.[2] On the following day, September 20th, the Florentine officers promptly responded with a letter of instructions which is exemplary in its precision and conciseness. In its almost telegraphic style one perceives the officers' concern to prevent misunderstanding, to avoid delays, to emphasize the need for precise and effective action:

you must straightway order that the persons of the family of the deceased be confined to the house. The household items used by the deceased must be separated from the others. You must bar the door of the house from the outside. The family of the deceased must receive victuals through the windows. Make sure that no one comes out. All members of the family have to be provided with victuals for the amount of one *giulio* per day. The money will be paid by the officer who pays the guards at the gates and it will be credited to him. All the above to be ordered and carried out at once. You will nform us of what follows.[3]

Unfortunately what followed was not good. With a letter dated October 2nd, 1630, the Health officers of Prato reported

1. ASF, *Sanità*, Copialettere, b. 55, c. 126 (11th Sept. 1630).
2. ASF, *Sanità*, Negozi, b. 150, c. 971.
3. ASF, *Sanità*, Copialettere, b. 55, c. 146 (20th Sept. 1630).

to the Board in Florence that the town was a prey to the plague.[1]

The first round of the battle had been lost. The invisible and pitiless enemy was within the walls claiming lives at a dreadful rate. People were religious and superstitious and they placed much faith in the Divine Providence. Although perfectly aware of how dangerous it was to gather in large groups, they organized processions and other religious ceremonies on October 8th, on October 28th and then again in November.[2] People however, were also practical and while stubbornly hoping for help from God or some other holy Dignitary, they knew that they had to help themselves in their own way.

There were two hospitals in Prato: the hospital *della Misericordia* and the hospital of San Silvestro, both of which were under the same administration. The governor was appointed by the Grand Duke and held office for a period of three years at the end of which he could be reappointed.[3] Over the centuries, these two hospitals had been endowed with property by various citizens and as their income was derived from such properties, their financial situation was largely dependent upon the level of agricultural prices. Around 1630, in normal years, the income of the two hospitals fluctuated around 5,500-7,500 ducats.[4] In a year of exceptionally low agricultural prices, such as 1634, the income of the two hospitals could drop as low as 2,500 ducats.[5]

1. ASF, *Sanità*, Copialettere, b. 55, c. 167v-168.
2. GIANI, *Pestilenze*, pp. 103-4.
3. ASP, *Diurno 2*, c. 175 (5th Dec. 1630).
4. ASP, *Fondo Comunale*, b. 587, cc. 1037-1041; 1043 ff.; 1058-1060; 1362 ff.
5. ASP, *Fondo Comunale*, b. 588, cc. 194 and 217.

The hospital regularly received patients for treatment, but this was only incidental. According to an old tradition of medieval origin, the hospitals of Prato like most European hospitals, were devoted to charity at large rather than to the specific task of attending the sick. Between July 1st, 1631 and June 30th, 1632 for example, the two hospitals received 292 patients for a total of 3,692 patient-days, which meant an average permanence of about 13 days per patient. This was approximately equivalent to having had 10 patients for the 365 days of the year. For the 365 days of the year the hospital *della Misericordia* kept 182 abandoned adolescents (128 girls and 54 boys)[1] and also cared for about 100 foundlings. Although the hospital had resident wet nurses, most of the foundlings were given out to non resident wet nurses who of course received compensation for their services. In 1630 the ratio of foundlings kept in the hospital to those given out was 8 to 98.[2] All the above figures conform with a normal pattern, and they clearly show that the vast majority of the resources of the two hospitals was devoted to the care of abandoned youth.

Normally Prato could also count on the services of a number of surgeons and physicians. Early in September 1630, the Health officers of Florence wanted to know the strength of the medical profession in Prato and complying with their request the administration of Prato reported the following:[3]

. . . The Community of Prato keeps two physicians as *medici condotti*. One is ser Latanzio Magiotti, aged about 40, bachelor, very

1. ASP, *Fondo Comunale*, b. 587, cc. 1058-1060. Among the foundlings girls always outnumbered boys. In 1552 in the *Hospital for Innocents* of Florence the ratio of girls to boys was even higher than in 1630 Prato, namely 900 girls against 300 boys (BATTARA, *Popolazione*, p. 34).

2. ASP, *Fondo Comunale*, b. 587, c. 1362 ff.

3. ASF, *Sanità*, Negozi, b. 150, c. 306 (6th Sept. 1630). See also *Sanità*, Negozi, b. 151, c. 600 (14th October 1630).

good doctor, patrician, native of Montevarchi.[1] The other is messer Giobatta Serrati, native of Castiglione Fiorentino, aged 30 with wife and one daughter and is a good doctor. Native of this place is messer Pierfrancesco Fabbruzzi, who has a private practice, is 70 years of age, married with children, a good doctor if he were not so old. In addition there is messer Giuliano Losti, a young man of 25 years of age. He obtained his doctorate in medicine this year and thus far has not put his knowledge into practice. There is also messer Jacopo Lionetti, aged 60, with wife and children who, however, has never practised.

Although you did not request information about either the quantity or quality of the surgeons, we inform you that there are three surgeons, two of which are in *condotta*: they are Master Michele Cepparelli, native of this place, aged 60, with great experience and without wife or children and Master Antonio Gramigna, native of this place, aged 50, with wife and children, one of whom is at present learning the art from his father. There is also Master Tiburzio,[2] native of this place, who has a private practice, aged 60 with wife and children.

It might be mentioned here that in Italy since the thirteenth century, first in the cities and later also in the villages of some importance, it had become customary to hire physicians and surgeons at the expense of the community. These physicians (and surgeons) were either called *medici* (and *chirurghi*) *condotti* or also *medici* (and *chirurghi*) *del pubblico*. Receiving a regular monthly salary they were to reside in the community, never to leave without permission and to cure without charge all

1. Ser Latanzio Magiotti was baptized in Montevarchi on June 27th, 1590 and received his doctorate at the University of Pisa in May 1612. In time he became famous and was appointed physician to the Grand Duke Ferdinand II. In 1636 Galileo was one of his patients (GALILEI, *Opere*, vol. 20, pp. 239 and 472).

2. This was Tiburzio Bardi, appointed surgeon of the pest-house in the hospital of San Silvestro on October 22nd, 1630. On the three surgeons, Gramigna, Cepparelli and Bardi, see also below pp. 51-2.

those in need of medical care who could not afford its cost. On occasion, when treating people of some means, they were allowed to receive an extra fee.[1] Besides these doctors and surgeons there were the physicians and surgeons with private practices. According to the report cited above, Prato had two physicians *condotti* and two physicians with private practice as well as one man who held a doctorate but never practised. Moreover, there were two surgeons *condotti* and one with private practice. This gives a grand total of seven active medical men for a population of about 17,000 souls, – definitely a high ratio for the time. Whether a relatively high number of doctors was beneficial to the health of the population is another matter.

When the plague broke out in the town, the ordinary medical structure of Prato had to be reorganized and strengthened. The Health officers of Prato informed the Board in Florence that their town was a prey of the plague on October 2nd; that same day they hurriedly decided to transform one of the two hospitals into a pest-house. Since the hospital *della Misericordia* housed the children, the officers selected the hospital of San Silvestro with the annexed church of San Silvestro. The hospital *della Misericordia* however, had to provide the

1. On the duties of the *medici condotti*, see ASP, *Fondo Bonamici*, b. 9 *Obblighi de medici condotti della Comunità di Prato*. Around 1630, the salary of these physicians was 700 *lire* per year. On top of the regular salary, each doctor received also an allowance of 126 *lire* a year for housing (ASP, *Fondo Comunale*, b. 1038). The surgeons *condotti* received only 16 *staia* of wheat and 10 *barili* of wine per year (on these measures see Appendix 2). In 1632 however the Town administration was unable to fill a vacancy and it was recognized that the inadequacy of the public salary was the reason. It was decided therefore to give the surgeons *condotti* a yearly salary of 24 ducats (= 168 *lire*) each (ASP, *Diurno* 3, c. 112v., 21st Jan. 1632).

hospital of San Silvestro with the food, the medicines, the fuel, the beds and the other equipment necessary to operate as a pest-house. The town was to cover the expenses for the personnel.[1]

The officers appointed a confessor, a surgeon and a number of attendants to serve in the pest-house. They also appointed gravediggers, guards, a messenger, a man to deliver the victuals to those confined in their homes and a man to carry the necessities from the hospital *della Misericordia* to the hospital of San Silvestro.[2] Including the physicians, the surgeons, the vice-chancellor who issued the passes, the gravediggers, the chief constable and his men, those who in one way or another fought the plague in Prato under the orders of the Health officers, numbered about twenty-five at the peak of their strength.[3]

The physicians were persons of rank. The surgeons were on a markedly lower social level. At one point, some of the guards at the gates were put in jail,[4] which proves that their conduct was not always exemplary. The gravediggers were an unpleasant and mercenary group[5] and the nicknames given to some of them clearly indicate vulgar and brutal people.[6] On one occasion we know that a convict was enlisted as a gravedigger because of lack of regular help.[7] This was the army

1. ASP, *Diurno* 2, c. 149 v. See also ASF, *Sanità*, Copialettere, b. 55, c. 167v-168.

2. See below, Appendix 1.   3. See below Appendix 1.

4. ASF, *Sanità*, Copialettere, b. 55, c. 96 (27th Aug. 1630).

5. According to the Health Board in Florence the gravediggers of Prato, although regularly paid by the Community, extracted money from the families of the deceased, asking as much as 2 *scudi* for each body that they took away: ASF, *Sanità*, Copialettere, b. 57, c. 68v. (15th April 1631).

6. One was nicknamed *Michelaccio*, another *Vaccaio*.

7. ASP, *Diurno* 3, c. 52 (5th Aug. 1631).

which the Health officers led in their fight against the plague – a small army and a very heterogeneous one, which included physicians as well as constables, friars as well as convicts.

It was not easy to keep this small army at full strength. The plague claimed lives among those who served the Public Health as well as among those who were served by it, and the details of this sad story are presented in Appendix 1.

Who were the Health officers? Normally they were prominent local people, persons of rank, *gentilhuomini*, possibly selected among those who had some experience with administration. When in September 1630 the Community of Fiorenzuola elected the local officers, it reported to the Board in Florence that 'they all are *gentilhuomini* of this community and they are people of means. Each one is head of a family with wife and children. They all reside permanently in this community'.[1]

In large towns such as Milan, the Health Board included a physician, but in general the Health officers had no medical background. It might be surprising but it was not absurd that people totally unacquainted with medical theory or practice would be appointed to such an office. In the main towns, the officers could consult with the College of Physicians for technical advice. The officers of the minor centres could consult with the local physicians, reported to the central Health officers of their respective capitals and received from the latter both instructions and information. Last but not least, much of the work of the Health officers was to issue ordinances and to establish controls regarding the confinement of people, the suspension of communications, the establishment and the

1. ASF, *Sanità*, Negozi, b. 150, c. 840 (16th Sept. 1630).

administration di pest-houses. Such business did not require direct personal knowledge of medical matters.

Cristofano di Giulio Ceffini, one of the Health officers of Prato, wrote a manuscript with the title *Libro della Sanità*. At one point in his book Cristofano gives a summary of what he believed a Public Health officer ought to know in time of plague:[1]

It has been proven by experience that to put down an epidemic, first of all it is necessary to resort to the Majesty of God and to the intercession of the Holy Virgin and of the Saints. Then it is necessary to observe with every possible diligence the following rules:
– to disinfect with sulphur and perfumes all homes or rooms wherein there has been death or sickness;
– to separate at once the sick from the healthy as soon as the case of illness is discovered;
– to burn and take away at once those objects such as have been used by the deceased or by the sick;
– to shut up straight away all houses wherein there have been infected people and keep them closed for at least 22 days so that those who are segregated inside the houses will not carry the infection to other people;
– to stop trade.

Most of this was common sense. A few technical items in the recipe such as the term of 22 days for the quarantine originated from the instructions sent out by the Magistrates of Florence.[2] Perusing the medical literature of the time one does not find much to add to the guidelines given by Cristofano. One only finds that there was no consensus of opinion about the limited

1. ASP, LS, c. 86v. On the *Libro della sanita* see below p. 65ff.
2. See below Appendix 8 and also ASF, *Sanità*, Copialettere b. 55, c. 9 (22nd June 1630).

quarantine of 22 days and it is worth noticing that Cristofano does not seem to have been aware of the debate.

Their technical knowledge may have been limited, but in a town infected by the plague, the work and the responsibilities that fell on the shoulders of the Health officers were immense. As the *Podestà* of Prato reported to Florence[1] the local officers met with him, in the *Palazzo*, every day, sometimes late in the evening, to deal with innumerable problems and never ending difficulties. People were reluctant to obey the orders; there were patients in the lararetto who did not even respect confinement and guards had to be provided for the pest-house.[2] About the middle of November the plague broke out in the prison.[3] Vigilance at the gates of the city was not always satisfactory: on November 14, at the suggestion of a Commissioner of the Health Board of Florence, it was decided to close all gates permanently with the exception of Porta Mercatale and Porta Pistoiese (see p. 39) and special guards had to be placed at these gates.[4] On November 23rd the plague broke out in the countryside[5] and this created a whole series of new difficulties.[6] In the meantime Pistoia, Florence and other Tuscan towns severed communications with Prato,[7] which began to suffer from shortage of necessities.[8] As the plague progressed there was more need for gravediggers and for attend-

1. ASF, *Sanità*, Negozi, b. 153, c. 973 (20th Dec. 1630).
2. ASP, *Diurno* 2, c. 171 (9th Nov. 1630).
3. ASF, *Sanità*, Negozi, b. 152, c. 611, 629, 1048.
4. ASP, *Diurno* 2, c. 171v.
5. ASF, *Sanità*, Negozi, b. 152, c. 1048.   6. See below, p. 102.
7. ASF, *Sanità*, Negozi, b. 151, c. 270 (6th Oct. 1630), c. 600v. (14th Oct. 1630); b. 152, c. 404 (9th Nov. 1630).
8. ASF, *Sanità*, Negozi, b. 152, c. 490 (11th Nov. 1630) and c. 610 (14th Nov. 1630).

ants in the pest-house. But the plague killed them too and the officers had to worry constantly about their replacement and their requests for higher wages.[1]

Surgeons, or at least people with some surgical training, presented a yet more serious problem. As we have seen above, when the plague broke out, beside the doctors, there were in Prato three surgeons, masters Gramigna and Cepparelli who were *condotti* and master Tiburzio who had a private practice and was later appointed to the pest-house in the hospital of San Silvestro.[2] However, on October 13th master Gramigna died.[3] On November 1st master Tiburzio died too.[4] Master Cepparelli had declared that he would not attend infected people, and as he was old and gave satisfactory service to the rest of the population, his attitude was tolerated.[5] Early in November 1630 he fell sick.[6] We do not know the nature of the disease but we do know he recovered and continued to refuse to treat the victims of the plague.[7] Thus Prato was without a surgeon for the infected. The officers had requested a new surgeon from Florence as early as October 8th when

1. See below Appendix 1.

2. ASP, *Diurno 2*, c. 161. The appointment was made on October 22nd, 1630.

3. ASF, *Sanità*, Negozi, b. 151, c. 600 (14th Oct. 1630). Master Gramigna died of 'a long illness' and therefore not of the plague. A letter from Prato to the Board in Florence dated Nov. 5th confirms that master Gramigna had died of 'ordinary illness' (ASF, *Sanità*, Negozi, b. 152, c. 210).

4. ASP, *Fondo Comunale*, b. 3081, *Morti Maschi e Femmine* from 1630 to 1648.

5. ASF, *Sanità*, Negozi, b. 151, c. 365 (8th Oct. 1630).

6. ASF, *Sanità*, Negozi, b. 152, c. 210 (5th Nov. 1630).

7. In 1634 Master Cepparelli still held his position of surgeon *condotto* (ASP, *Fondo Comunale*, b. 588, c. 292). He died on July 30th, 1646 (ASP, *Fondo Comunale*, b. 3081, *Morti Maschi e Femmine* from 1630 to 1648). The Michele Cepparelli who died on November 11th, 1630 (ASP, *Fondo Comunale*, b. 3081) was not our surgeon.

master Gramigna was sick and the officers were afraid that he would die.[1] On November 5th. after the death of master Tiburzio and with master Cepparelli sick, the officers renewed their request in tones of urgency.[2] Unfortunately the Board in Florence was in no position to help: 'We suffer from a great lack of surgeons,' they wrote, 'and despite our diligence we do not seem able to secure enough of them. Try to find one and bring him to Prato with a just salary'.[3] The suggestion was unrealistic and it was expressed only to keep alive a flame of hope in the hearts of the officers in Prato. If the Board of Florence who controlled the situation in the whole Grand Duchy was unable to find a surgeon, how could the poor officers of Prato, confined to their town under what amounted to conditions of siege, hope to succeed in the task? They did not; and to understand the gravity of the situation, one has to consider that while the care offered by the physicians had only a psychological value, the surgeon by lancing a festering bubo could alleviate excruciating pain and give the impression of speeding up the recovery of the patient. That in Prato surgical attendance was no longer available for the infected was regarded as an 'iniquitous fact'.

Another very difficult problem that kept bothering the heads of the officers was that of the pest-house.

As time went on and the plague ravaged the town, it became clearer and clearer that keeping the pest-house within the walled area had been a tragic mistake. Despite the guards put at the gate of the pest-house, it was practically impossible to keep the sick in complete isolation. The pest-house had to be

1. ASF, *Sanità*, Negozi b. 151, c. 365.
2. ASF, *Sanità*, Negozi b. 152, c. 210.
3. ASF, *Sanità*, Copialettere b. 56, c. 27 (9th Nov. 1630).

moved outside the walls, but where? The Health Board of Florence sent commissioner Coveri to Prato to assist the local officers, but instead of making things easier the arrival of Coveri further complicated the matter. He and the officers of Prato could hardly agree on anything. According to the Pratesi the most suitable place to serve as a pest-house was the Convent of St Anne, half a mile from Prato (see p. 39). According to the commissioner the rooms on the main floor of the Convent were too damp. Coveri's choice was a building called *il Palco* which belonged to another religious community, the *Padri Zoccolanti*, and was situated at the other end of the town's territory. For the convalescents he suggested the requisition of a villa that belonged to the Florentine family of the Ghori. The officers of Prato agreed on the choice of the villa but they strongly opposed the choice of *il Palco*. They rightly pointed out that the place was much too far from the town and it could only be reached by a difficult road. The *Podestà* who was one of the officers *ex officio* agreed with his colleagues. As he reported to Florence, even the healthy, let alone the sick, could hardly have withstood the hardships or being moved from Prato to *il Palco* in mid-winter.[1]

The friars themselves were behind the dispute, as each religious community tried to put on the other the unpleasant burden and the discomfort of having its convent turned into a pest-house. The *Padri Zoccolanti* expressed their opposition in strong and direct terms. They accused Coveri of collusion with the Fathers of St Anne – 'Coveri had dinner with them . . .'[2] – and declared that they would yield only to an order from the Grand Duke. Even with such an order they would leave the convent only under nine conditions which they formally pre-

1. For all the preceding points, see ASF, *Sanità*, Negozi, b. 152, c. 611-29 (14th Nov. 1630) and c. 816 and 831 (18th Nov. 1630).

2. ASF, *Sanità*, Negozi, b. 152, c. 571 (13th Nov. 1630).

sented in writing.[1] The fathers of St Anne used more subtle tactics. They turned to the Grand Duke and reminded him that in 1512, when the Medici cardinal who later became Pope Leo X moved against Florence leading Spanish troops, he took up residence at the Convent of St Anne. While he was there, the Pratesi aimed their fire at the Convent and the future Pope was saved thanks to the intercession of the miraculous Virgin in the Church of the Convent. The tactful friars did not mention that on that occasion the troops of the Cardinal ruthlessly sacked Prato. Instead they reminded the Grand Duke that out of gratitude for the hospitality of the friars and for the intercession of the miraculous Virgin, through his nephew – also a Medici and also a Cardinal – Pope Leo granted the friars full immunity from the jurisdiction of the Pratesi, who had acted nastily and oppressively toward them ever since. In conclusion the fathers petitioned the Grand Duke to confirm the privileges granted by his ancestors and not to allow the convent to be converted into a pest-house.[2]

The Grand Duke was not impressed by the petition and the miraculous Virgin was probably too busy with other matters. Yet for a moment it seemed as if the views of Coveri would prevail. The officers in Prato did not have a high opinion of Coveri[3] but they respected the Board that he represented and they thought that he carried great authority in Florence. Consequently, tired of the long discussions and of the delays that the discussions caused, they were ready to accept the solu-

1. ASF, *Sanità*, Negozi, b. 152, c. 611-629 (14th Nov. 1630).
2. ASF, *Sanità*, Negozi, b. 152, c. 698 (15th Nov. 1630).
3. In a letter dated 18th Nov. 1630 addressed to the Board in Florence the *Podestà* of Prato wrote of Coveri that 'you (the officers of Florence) told us that he is an intelligent person', obviously implying that he and the officers in Prato held a different view (ASF, *Sanità*, Negozi, b. 152, c. 816 and 831).

tion proposed by the Commissioner. But at this point, a new
fact intervened. According to Coveri's plan, a villa of the
Ghori was to be requisitioned to house the convalescents. The
Ghori were an influential family in Florence. As soon as they
became aware of what was being planned in Prato, they
swiftly contacted their powerful acquaintances. On November
15th, the Health Board in Florence wrote to Prato that there
were also villas belonging to the citizens of Prato which would
be suitable as pest-houses and the like, and that it did not seem
right that the Pratesi 'should be exempt and the Florentine
burdened for a matter which was to benefit Prato . . . For this
reason you will order that the Florentine landlords should go
unmolested'.[1] The tone of the letter was strong, and the letter
itself showed the Pratesi that Coveri was after all a man with
little authority. When he next appeared at a meeting in Prato
imperiously informing the officers and the *Podestà* that the
Board in Florence expected them to immediately transfer the
pest-house to the *Palco*, his words were brushed aside. The
Officers decided to use the Convent of St Anne as the pest-
house and *il Palco* as the convalescent-home.[2] The decision
was taken on the 17th or the 18th of November and on
November 20th it was endorsed by the Board in Florence.[3]
Nine days later, on the evening of Friday 29th, a new Commissioner of the Board arrived in Prato. The same night, he
had a meeting with the *Podestà* and the officers, and the following day they all visited the Convent of St Anne, the *Palco* and
many other places in the countryside.[4] The new Commissioner
agreed fully with all that the officers of Prato had done and

1. ASF, *Sanità*, Copialettere, b. 56, c. 39v.
2. ASF, *Sanità*, Negozi, b. 152, c. 816 and 831 (18th Nov. 1630).
3. ASF, *Sanità*, Copialettere, b. 56, c. 44-44v.
4. ASF, *Sanità*, Negozi, b. 153, c. 93 (2nd Dec. 1630) and c. 973 (20th
Dec. 1630).

gave his blessing to their decisions. The thorny question of the pest-house seemed settled at last. But it was not. It soon became clear that the Convent of St Anne and *il Palco* were too far apart and that it was unthinkable to transfer convalescents from one place to the other in the middle of the winter. But where were the convalescents to be housed? A frantic new search was launched and eventually the officers concluded that if the pest-house was to be in the Convent of St Anne as already decided, the ideal place for the convalescents was a villa that belonged to Lattanzio Vai near the Convent. We have every reason to believe that this was a reasonable and honest choice. But Lattanzio Vai was a very important person; he was a canon and a member of a prominent and wealthy family of Prato. Probably the officers counted on the fact that Prato was 'banished' and the Pratesi were not allowed to go to Florence or to send letters there. Perhaps they also underestimated the influence of don Lattanzio.

During the month of December the officers had managed to find a house in Prato for the fathers of St Anne,[1] and they had moved the belongings of the friars from the convent into the annexed church, which was closed and walled up.[2] Beds, mattresses, pots, pans and other goods had also been brought from the hospital *della Misericordia* to the Convent of St Anne. This had not been an easy operation because the administration of the hospital was reluctant to provide the necessary equip-

1. ASF, *Sanità*, Negozi, b. 153, c. 731 and 744 (14th Dec. 1630); ASP, *Diurno* 3, c. 164v. (2nd Sept. 1632). The fathers of St Anne never stopped complaining: early in December they protested that the building in which they were housed was inadequate because of 'the small number' and the 'poor quality' of the rooms (ASF, *Sanità*, Copialettere, b. 56, c. 68, 4th Dec. 1630).

2. ASP, LS, c. 58v. The reason for this was to protect the belongings of the Fathers from contagion.

ment, but the officers did their best to obtain all they could. On December 31st, the *Podestà* of Prato wrote to the Health Board in Florence that 'the new pest-house at St Anne is in order . . . and two days hence we will start transferring those who are now in the pest-house in Prato'.[1] The *Podestà* did not know that the very same day don Lattanzio was writing a petition to the Board in Florence. In the petition don Lattanzio stated that he lived in the villa that the Health officers of Prato were ready to requisition, that he had no other place to move to, and that it was a great injustice to dislodge him when so many other buildings were available.[2] In all likelihood, don Lattanzio had powerful friends in Florence and they immediately came to his support. With a letter dated January 1st, 1631 the Board in Florence warned the officers in Prato not to bother don Lattanzio and not to requisition his villa.[3]

There are moments in life when one is under the impression that the Prince of Darkness is taking his due and something over. When the letter of the Board reached the Officers in Prato such may well have been their feeling. More than two long months of exacting efforts, lengthy discussions and great expenses were in danger of being totally wasted. The *Podestà* took up his pen and answered Florence with a very strong letter throwing all the weight of his influence in support of his colleagues. The tone of his letter gives an idea of the mood in Prato. The *Podestà* openly accused don Lattanzio of lying. Don Lattanzio was not living in the villa but in Prato. It was not true that he had no other places in which to live because he owned two houses in Prato and three other villas in the countryside. It was not true that there were many other buildings close to the Convent of St Anne that could easily be used

1. ASF, *Sanità*, Negozi, b. 153, c. 1358.
2. ASF, *Sanità*, Negozi, b. 153, c. 153 (31st Dec. 1630).
3. ASF, *Sanità*, Copialettere, b. 56, c. 117.

for convalescents. The letter of the *Podestà* ends on a very firm note: 'The decision to requisition the villa was taken only under pressure of great necessity. You must believe this, because to displease an important person is not done unless one is forced to it. Sirs, this is a very necessary measure'.[1]

If the letter of the Board had caused consternation in Prato, the letter of the *Podestà* caused no less embarrassment in Florence. The Board did not answer and its silence implicitly meant that the Pratesi had to find a solution and to settle their quarrels. They did. The fathers of St Anne owned a house in the vicinity of their convent with some property attached which was surrounded by a wall and was thus called *'la casa del poder murato'* (see p. 39). The Fathers allowed the town to use this house for the convalescents. In compensation for this extra burden the wealthy don Lattanzio made a donation to the Friars which no doubt entitled him to a place in paradise and enabled him to retain his villa for his own use.[2]

Now at last everything was settled for the transfer of the pest-house from the hospital of San Silvestro to the Convent of St Anne. On January 13th, 1631 the officers appointed Diacinto Gramigna to serve in the new pest-house as surgeon-attend-ant.[3] Diacinto was the son of the late master Gramigna and had learned some rudiments of surgery from working with his father. He was not a fully trained surgeon but the officers had been searching for a surgeon for months and always in vain. Thus they not only appointed the young Gramigna; they also granted him a generous salary.[4] On January 14th, in the middle of the harsh Tuscan winter, forty-three inmates of the hospital

1. ASF, *Sanità*, Negozi, b. 154, c. 61 (2nd Jan. 1631).

2. ASP, LS, c. 58v.

3. ASP, *Diurno* 2, c. 184 v. Diacinto, however, did not take up service until February 16th.

4. See below, Appendix 1.

of San Silvestro were moved to the new pest-house at the Convent of St Anne. It must have been a sad, awe-inspiring procession. But none of the forty-three sufferers died that day nor in the two days following.[1]

Conflicts, abuses and infringements of regulations, petty quarrels, and a never-ending series of problems and difficulties – every day the Health officers had to face such things, while indefatigable vigilance was required and the bells of the churches kept announcing new deaths. What did these eight men feel deep in their hearts?

A sense of intolerable fatigue and constant worry is frequently mentioned in the correspondence. A revealing notation discloses that on occasion some officers fell prey to the loneliness and selfquestioning which sensitive men feel when in a position of ultimate responsibility at a time of tragic crisis:

one learns at the cost of human life what happens when one receives from God the scourge of an epidemic without having any light or experience wherewith to guide one's conduct in so exacting a task.[2]

A third theme in the psychological history of the Health officers of Prato is a desperate sense of frustration. At one point in his book of notes, Cristofano Ceffini wrote:[3]

The epidemic started in the month of August 1630, slowly at first so that people took no notice of its gathering momentum, thinking that any day it would end. In truth people went about their business and took little account of what was beginning to happen

1. ASP, LS, cc. 58v.-59.

2. This notation appears on the lower part of the first page of the *Libro della Sanità* by Cristofano Ceffini but was written by a different hand. On the *Libro della Sanità* by Cristofano Ceffini see below p. 65.

3. ASP, LS, c. 67v.

because they had no experience of such a catastrophe.

Health officers may be too exacting when they demand scrupulous obedience to certain rules; on the other hand, it is all too easy for people to act foolishly and dismiss sound advice. The people of Prato were no exception. As far as grape production went, 1630 was a vintage year with an abundant harvest.[1] In September and October, many Pratesi insisted on moving to the village of Tavola to pick the grapes when the village had already been 'closed' because of a number of suspicious deaths and illnesses.[2] I have already mentioned that despite all precautions it was difficult to keep the inmates of the pest-house in complete isolation.[3] On October 8th, the Health officers of Prato desperately reported 'that their orders are scarcely respected and their ordinances hardly obeyed, hence their work is almost totally frustrated'.[4] From the Grand Duke they requested an edict contemplating capital punishment for the transgressors. Their request was accepted[5] but they did not really intend to apply the ordinance and things went on as before. When the Commissioner of the Health Board in Florence, Signor Cavalier Francesco Vincenzo Martelli inspected Prato at the end of November he found 'a most unsatisfactory situation. They have the pest-house within the city . . . the sick often leave the pest-house and communicate with other people. This lack of discipline is of such proportions that the city is suffering badly from the disease'.[6]

1. GALILEO, *Opere*, vol. 14, p. 135.
2. ASF, *Sanità*, Copialettere, b. 55, c. 137v. (7th Sept. 1630), c. 167v. (3rd Oct. 1630) and *Sanità*, Negozi, b. 150 (29th Sept. 1630).
3. See above p. 50.   4. ASF, *Sanità*, Negozi, b. 151, c. 365.
5. ASF, *Sanità*, Copialettere, b. 56, c. 27 (9th Nov. 1630).
6. ASF, *Sanità*, Negozi, b. 153, c. 100 ff. The report is undated but it is among letters dated December 2nd, 1630. The pest-house was moved out of town on the following January 14th.

Signor Martelli arrived in Prato late in the evening of Friday November 29th. He spent most of the following Saturday visiting the countryside on horseback and inspecting the Convent of St Anne, the *Palco* and 'many other places' in search of the best possible location for the new pest-house. He left Prato late on the same Saturday.[1] Signor Martelli could not have had the opportunity of observing the infringements and abuses that he reported. His report obviously echoed the complaints of the officers. In fact in their discussions the officers and signor Martelli had not only reached the decision to establish the new pest-house in the Convent of St Anne but to put an end to the 'most unsatisfactory situation', they also had agreed to create a new office, that of *Provveditore della Sanità*. Whether the idea originated from the officers or from the Commissioner the documents do not say, but they do say that the step 'was necessary'. One of the officers was to be appointed to the new position. The *Provveditore* would not supplant the other officers, either in their authority or in their function to set forth ordinances in the matter of Public Health. The *Provveditore* would take upon himself the responsibility for the correct, prompt, and accurate execution of the decisions of the officers and he would ensure the proper functioning of all services connected with Public Health: in other words he would be the executive arm of the officers. Because of the importance, responsibility and extent of the work, it was thought that the office must be remunerated.[2]

On December 11th, 1630, ten days after the visit of Commissioner Martelli, the Health officers met for the election of

1. ASF, *Sanità*, Negozi, b. 153, c. 93 (2nd Dec. 1630) and c. 973 (20th Dec. 1630).
2. See below, p. 116, n. 1.

the *Provveditore*. A unanimous vote elected Cristofano di Giulio Ceffini.[1]

Cristofano came from an untitled but prominent family of Prato. Francesco di Bartolomeo di Francesco appears in the tax poll of 1480. He had two sons, Sebastian and Francesco. From Francesco, Giulio was born and from Giulio, Cristofano.[2]

In the list of those who paid the predial tithe in 1621 Giulio di Francesco is taxed a little more than 6 florins. This put him thirtieth in the list. All those who were taxed 5 florins and above were definitely among the well-off. The richest were taxed 18 florins. Giulio was thus in the lower group of the wealthy landowners.[3] A typical member of the oligarchies that ruled the Communities of the Grand Duchy, Cristofano had a strong bent for public administration, and he frequently stood for election. On the first of March 1629 he was elected *Gonfaloniere* of Prato, thus reaching the highest elective office in town.[4] With the eight *Priori*, a *Gonfaloniere* remained in office for the term of two months, thus Cristofano's *Gonfalonierato* terminated on April 30th. On August 14th, he was appointed member of the commission for the selection of the community physician.[5] From September 1st to the end of October he was one of the *Priori*.[6] On October 27th, he was appointed substitute *Provveditore di Palazzo*, a

1. ASP, *Diurno* 2, c. 176v.
2. For all this see FIUMI, *Prato*, p. 344.
3. FIUMI, *Prato*, pp. 197-8.   4. ASP, *Diurno* 2, c. 98.
5. ASP, *Diurno* 2, c. 49v. The Commission presented its report and conclusions on August 30th (*Ibid.*, c. 52).
6. ASP, *Diurno* 2, c. 139v. (1st Sept. 1630), and *Fondo Comunale* 1038, c. 62.

position that placed him in charge of military provision.[1] It was in this role of Provveditore di Palazzo that, a few days after taking office, Cristofano advised the Health officer of Prato to place the border guards at the *Passo della Cerbaia* rather than at the *Passo dell'Antella*, a suggestion that was praised and accepted because it meant less expense and more efficient control.[2] On December 31st, Cristofano stood for the office of *Provveditore della Comunità*, but this time he failed.[3] On August 3rd, 1630, when the number of the Health officers was raised from four to eight, he was appointed as one of them.[4] At this juncture, with the plague on the doorstep, other prominent citizens refused such an appointment, which carried with it risky responsibilities and no remuneration. As the town council remarked 'one sees the difficulty of finding a person who would accept',[5] but it does not seem that Cristofano hesitated a moment in accepting the office. His civic sense and his passion for public administration were all too genuine and deep rooted. It is not surprising that on December 11th, 1630, tired, worried, and frustrated, badly needing someone both firm and competent to handle people and money, the Health officers of Prato appointed Cristofano to the office of *Provveditore della Sanitá*.

As far as I know Cristofano had never studied medicine. By training and inclination he was a clerk and accountant.[6]

1. ASP, *Diurno* 2, c. 68.   2. See above p. 37, n. 3.
3. ASP, *Diurno* 2, c. 85v.   4. ASP, *Diurno* 2, c. 133v.
5. ASP, *Diurno* 2, c. 135v. and 136v. (16th Aug. 1630).
6. In April 1627 Cristofano applied for the position of scrivener of the *Opera del Cingolo*, a wealthy religious institution (ASP, *Fondo Comunale*, b. 587, c. 904). In 1628 he was appointed as one of the accountants who audited the accounts of another pious institution, the *Opera della Santissima Madonna del Soccorso fuori Prato* (ASP, *Fondo Comunale*, b. 587, c. 1448). In May 1630 he was one of the two accountants who audited the books of the town administration (ASP, *Diurno* 2, c. 120). In 1630-32 Cristofano was

I have already indicated that in those days it was not considered necessary to be a medical man in order to be a Public Health officer.[1] When Cristofano was appointed *Provveditore della Sanità* his duties were carefully specified:[2]

First. He must take precautions so as to keep both the pest-house and the convalescent home well provided with all necessary provisions; to keep a sharp eye open for negligences; and to make sure that the sick be brought to the pest-house.

Second. He must take precautions to isolate contacts in their homes and to ensure that subsidies are paid to them.

Third. He is responsible for the opening of the quarantined houses after the due period of isolation, provided that the necessary precautions are taken.

Fourth. He must enforce all decisions taken by the Health officers.

Fifth. He must carefully ensure that the Treasurer pays no more subsidies than there are people entitled to receive them; thus he must keep a vigilant eye on the distributors of the subsidies and report when the number of subsidized people diminishes because of death or other accident.

Sixth. He must look after those who are employed in the Public Health service and make sure that they carry out their duties; that both the sick and the convalescent are well treated and that the deceased are properly buried, and other such things.

It was a good list, the responsibilities were many and the salary was certainly not adequate. The officers and the *Podestà* had proposed a monthly salary of 8 ducats – the salary of a

administrator of the *Compagnia della disciplina* (ASP, *Fondo Comunale*, b. 588, c. 1257). After 1632 he was scrivener and accountant of the hospitals *della Misericordia* and of San Silvestro (ASP, *Fondo Comunale*, b. 588, c. 1043, 1076 and 1087).

1. See above p. 48.   2. ASP, *Diurno* 2, c. 176v. (11th Dec. 1630).

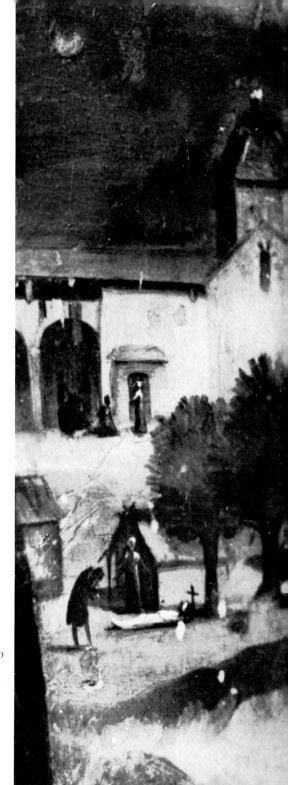

A common scene in the lazaretto of St Anne during the epidemic of 1630

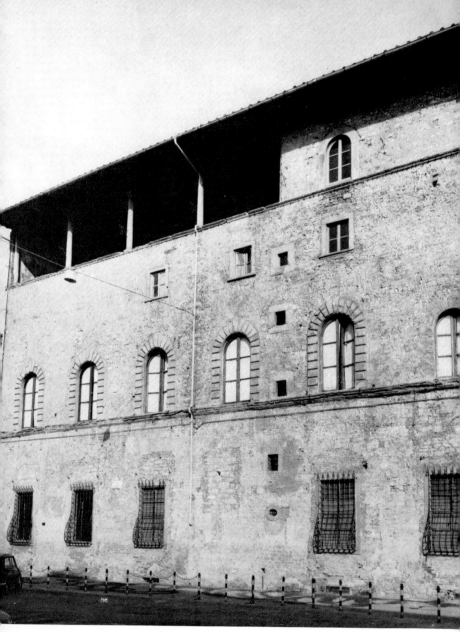

The hospital *della Misericordia* in Prato

gravedigger.[1] The fact is that the community expected prominent citizens to show civic sense and act by it. Somehow the
rule still held that *noblesse oblige*.

In the case of the *Provveditore della Sanità*, the sheer amount
of work to be done did not perhaps represent the major
challenge. It was not only a question of how much had to be
done but also, and even more, of *how* it was to be done. It was
necessary to act with the conviction that to tolerate infringements of the law meant to risk greater disaster, and yet it was
essential to temper the rigors of the law with humanity; it
was imperative to be strict in fighting abuses and to cut out
waste and at the same time it was necessary to show charity
and compassion. This implied the ability to keep a cool head,
a warm heart and a balanced judgement in a nightmare en-
vironment of death, misery and fear.

1. On the question of the salary of the *Provveditore* see below, p. 116, n. 1.

A PUZZLING INTERLUDE

In a petition addressed to the town administration, probably in 1634 or 1635, Cristofano states in the third person that:

at the time of the plague he was one of the Health officers and also *Provveditore*. All ordinances and measures taken passed through his hands and for his own satisfaction he kept a book in which he noted all events of those calamitous times. As he later showed this book to the Health officers, Morelli the *Podestà* and Mainardi the Chancellor asked him to make a copy of it to be deposited in the chancery for the common good.[1]

By inclination and proficiency, Cristofano was an account-ant and he filled his *Libro della Sanità* with figures. He gives the daily number of deaths from October 1st, 1630 to November 30th, 1631. He states the number of houses 'closed' because of infection, the number of people who lived within and received the subsidy, and the number of houses 'opened' because of termination of the quarantine. About the pest-house he reports daily the number of admissions, discharges, deaths and the number of the in-patients. Cristofano gives also figures about the items burned and those disinfected, about donations and expenses. All is presented with great precision, order and clarity. Hardly any mistake can be found in the numerous arithmetical operations involved.[2] For a social historian with a bent for quantitative analysis, the *Libro della Sanità* closely

1. ASP, *Fondo Comunale*, b. 588, c. 680 (the document is not dated).
2. Only in the accounts relating to the convalescents does one find dis-crepancies between the number of those who were dismissed from the hospital as convalescents and those who entered the convalescent-home. But it may be that not all those who left the hospital went into the con-

approaches what he imagines only in the rosiest of his dreams. But statistics rarely turn out to be a rosy affair.

In Prato, besides Cristofano, there were at least two other officials with a bent for figures. One of them was Giulio Morelli, appointed *Podestà* of Prato about the middle of November 1630. His predecessor never cared to send statistics to the Board in Florence, but the new *Podestà* was obviously eager to impress the Florentine authorities. From November 21st to December 31st, 1630, he regularly included daily figures on the deaths in Prato in all his letters.[1] Judging from his correspondence Giulio Morelli was a conscientious and competent official.

In Table 1 the daily figures given by Giulio Morelli are compared with those given by Cristofano Ceffini. Glancing at the Table the reader will realize that it is easier to write history when there are no statistics than when there are too many. At first the two sets of figures look hopelessly contradictory and the disagreement is even more surprising if one considers that the *Podestà* and Cristofano, as two of the eight Health officers, met practically every day, regularly exchanged information, and, as declared by Cristofano, the *Podestà* saw his *Libro* and praised it.

The disagreement is greater for the period following the first twelve days of December than for the preceding period. From November 21st to December 12th, Cristofano gives a

---

valescent-home and it is not impossible that some of those who entered the convalescent-home had been sick in their homes and not in the pest-house.

A minor discrepancy I have come across in the *Libro* is between the payment of 7 *lire* registered on c. 56v. for two palliasses as against 6 *lire* declared in c. 30v.

1. The letters are preserved in ASF, *Sanità*, Negozi, bb. 152 and 153.

TABLE I

Number of deaths in Prato according to different sources

Date		According to		Date		According to	
		Cristofano Ceffini	The Podestà			Cristofano Ceffini	The Podestà
Nov.	21	7	7	Dec.	11	4	3
	22	10	14		12	14	14
	23	11	9		13	10	5
	24	11	5		14	16	5
	25	10	3		15	7	8
	26	15	14		16	0	7
	27	14	13		17	11	3
	28	9	6		18	3	7
	29	10	12		19	0	6
	30	14	11		20	10	6
					21	12	4
Dec.	1	6	6		22	4	6
	2	3	5		23	2	2
	3	15	10		24	1	3
	4	6	9		25	3	7
	5	9	6		26	2	3
	6	2	7		27	9	7
	7	14	6		28	13	5
	8	10	10		29	9	3
	9	3	5		30	3	2
	10	10	5		31	2	0
				Total		324	269

total of 207 deaths, while the *Podestà* gives a total of 180, namely 13 per cent less. From December 13th to December 31st, Cristofano gives a total of 117 deaths, while the *Podestà* gives a total of 89, namely 24 per cent less. Moreover, from November 21st to December 12th the correlation coefficient between the two series has a value of 0.582 while for the subsequent period the value is 0.098. The Student t test shows these values significant at the level of 1 per cent. This indicates a statistically significant correlation before December 13th and a lack of significant correlation for the following period.[1] The epidemic subsided in the early part of December and it declined more markedly precisely after the middle of the month (see fig. 4).

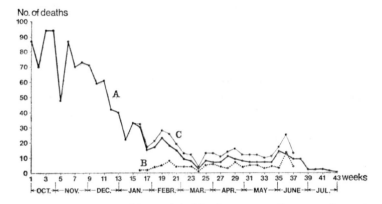

FIGURE 4. *Weekly totals of deaths as given by Cristofano*

    A   in the town of Prato.
    B   in the pest-house at St Anne.
    C   total of A+B.

From all these intricate comparisons and calculations one would conclude that while Cristofano reported all deaths in Prato, the *Podestà* reported only those deaths due to plague; but, however reasonable, this conclusion is untenable. On c. 82 of his *Libro*, giving the monthly summaries of deaths in Prato, Cristofano explicitly writes: 'Summary of deaths from contagion. Others have not been recorded.'

1. The Z transformation of the two correlation coefficients gives a normalized difference of 1.94 with $P \propto =0.052$ proving that the difference between the two coefficients is systematic.

This is not the end of the puzzle. On July 11th, 1631 the Town Council noted that 'for twenty-two days there have not been cases of infection nor deaths from contagion' and consequently it asked Florence to lift the ban of Prato.[1] Cristofano's statistics are not in agreement with this statement either. They mention 2 deaths on both June 23rd and June 24th and 1 death on both July 6th and July 7th.

Was Cristofano persistently exaggerating the ordeals of his town or were the other authorities minimizing the tragedy? I believe that no one wanted to suppress the truth, but truth has a way of shifting under pressure of opinions and interests. At a time when microbiological knowledge was non-existent, there were during an epidemic numerous deaths of dubious diagnosis. Cristofano wrote the *Libro* for 'his own satisfaction'. He had no interest in minimizing the tragedy and with his typical, almost pedantic precision, while recording the 'deaths from contagion' in all likelihood he took account also of the doubtful cases. When the *Podestà* reported the situation to Florence and the Town Council requested the lifting of the ban, they had no reasons for mentioning the 'suspicious deaths'. No one lied, but doubtful cases could easily be either counted or ignored. The hypothesis is not absurd and deserves to be pursued.

According to the official correspondence between the Health Board in Florence and Prato, 'suspicious cases' had occurred in Prato in late August and in the early part of September 1630, but plague was officially recognized for the first time on September 19th. Instead Cristofano twice states in his *Libro*[2] that the plague had started in August. Obviously Cristofano considered as plague also those cases which for the official records were only 'suspicious'. In view of the meticulous character of Cristofano, the fact is not surprising and if one

1. ASP, *Diurno* 3, c. 45.   2. ASP, LS, foreword and c. 67v.

looks at the curve of mortality in Prato (p. 69), judging from the typical shape of the epidemiological curves, one could hardly disagree with Cristofano's interpretation. Furthermore, according to the official version the epidemic was over by the end of June. But Cristofano still reports 5 deaths in July, 4 in August, 3 in September, 6 in October, 5 in November. Twenty-three deaths in five months for a population of about

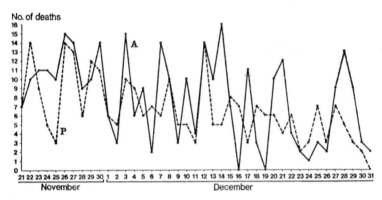

FIGURE 5. *Daily number of deaths in the town of Prato*
A as given by Cristofano.   P as given by the Podestà.

4,500 people (approximately those remaining in Prato after the plague) are equivalent to a mortality rate of 12 per thousand per year. The rate is too low to include deaths from all causes in a pre-industrial society. On the other hand, 8 houses were closed for quarantine in July, 3 in August, 2 in September and 5 in October,[1] which proves that endemically the plague was still present and 'suspicious' deaths kept occurring in the town. All available evidence points to one conclusion. As Cristofano states, he recorded only the deaths 'due to contagion'. However, he counted as deaths 'due to contagion' also those cases which being 'doubtful' were not officially reported

1. See Appendix 6.

to Florence although they caused locally the adoption of preventive health measures.

All this seems plausible and goes far to explain the discrepancies between the statistics of Cristofano and those of the *Podestà* but the puzzle is not completely solved. There still remains a mystery: for several days the number of deaths as given by the *Podestà* is higher than that given by Cristofano.

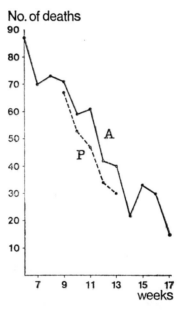

FIGURE 6. *Weekly totals of deaths in the town of Prato*
A as given by Cristofano.   P as given by the Podestà.
Number of weeks correspond to those in Fig. 4 (p. 69).

If instead of concentrating on the daily data and their absolute levels, one looks for the trend of mortality on the basis of weekly totals, one finds that the two series of Cristofano and the *Podestà* are related and indeed reveal the same trend (see fig. 6). Especially at the time when the epidemic was rampant a large number of cases of confirmed infection obviously gave the two series their common traits. The difference between the overall total of deaths given by Cristofano and that given by the *Podestà* for the period from 21st November to 31st December 1630 amounts to 55 deaths. Over the total given by Cristofano they represent about 17 per cent. The figure may be assumed as a rough index of the incertitude that prevailed in determining the cause of death in time of contagion.

The count of those who died in town was essentially given as statistical information for the benefit of both the local administrators and the authorities in Florence. Other health statistics had to be compiled in relation to administrative responsibilities. Cristofano had to oversee the distribution of the subsidy to those who were confined in their homes, thus he had to know daily how many houses were closed and how many people were confined in them. After the establishment of the pest-house in the Convent of St Anne, the hospital *della Misericordia* delivered the victuals to the lazaretto against a certificate with which every morning Cristofano reported the number of the patients in the pest-house and of the convalescents in the convalescent-home. Thus Cristofano had to keep close check of the movements of people in the two establishments. Faithfully and orderly he reported all these data in his *Libro della Sanità*.

Occasionally the *Podestà* sent to Florence quantitative information on various events pertaining to Public Health besides mortality. The following is a summary of his reports:

23rd November 1630[1]	in the pest-house	104 patients
14th December 1630[2]	in the pest-house	60 patients
		32 convalescents

1. ASF, *Sanità*, Negozi, b. 152, c. 1048.
2. ASF, *Sanità*, Negozi, b. 153, c. 731 and 744.

	sick in their homes	12 to 15
	houses quarantined	31
31st December 1630[1]	in the pest-house	60 persons sick and convalescent
25th February 1631[2]	in the pest-house	44 patients
	in the convalescent-home	5 convalescents

Most of the above data refer to a period for which Cristofano provides no information because either he had not yet been appointed *Provveditore* or the infected and convalescent were still housed in one of the two hospitals in Prato. At three points, however, the *Podestà*'s figures can be checked against Cristofano's, namely the information that on December 14th 1630 there were in Prato 31 houses closed, and that on February 25th 1631 there were 44 patients in the pest-house and 5 convalescents in the convalescent-home. According to Cristofano on December 14th, 1630 there were 58 houses closed and on February 25th, 1631 there were 49 patients in the pest-house and 5 convalescents in the convalescent-home. Thus there is perfect agreement between the *Podestà* and Cristofano about the number of convalescents on February 25th. There is a quasi-agreement about the number of patients in the pest-house at the same date. There is a quite considerable disagreement about the number of houses closed on December 14th. All this is puzzling enough, although the details given by Cristofano about the houses closed induce one to believe that if there was one who was mistaken, it was the *Podestà*.

Besides Cristofano and the *Podestà* there was one other official with a liking for figures, Vincenzo Mainardi, the

1. ASF, *Sanità*, Negozi, b. 153, c. 1358.
2. ASF, *Sanità*, Negozi, b. 155, cc. 813 and 820.

Chancellor of Prato. On February 5th, 1631, in a letter addressed to the Health Board in Florence, the Chancellor reported that there were:[1]

in the pest-house	43 patients
in the convalescent-home	14 convalescents
houses quarantined	20 with 45 persons confined in them

All this agrees admirably with the information supplied by
Cristofano.

A final remark. In 1635 two accountants appointed by the
Community of Prato audited the accounts of all expenditure
for Public Health over the previous years. The two accountants
were Lapo di Messer Piero Migliorati and Francesco di
Giovanni Geppi and among other accounts they audited also
the accounts of Cristofano Ceffini. They carefully inspected the
Libro della Sanità, did not notice any mistake or fraud and
accepted the evidence of the *Libro* at face value.[2]

I apologize to the reader for this boringly technical interlude.
Although puzzled by the discrepancies between some of the
figures given by Cristofano and the figures given by the
Podestà, I feel that I can proceed with my story relying on
Cristofano with cautious confidence, strengthened by the
example of the two accountants Francesco di Giovanni and
Lapo di Messer Piero.

1. ASF, *Sanità*, Negozi, b. 155, c. 261 and 280.
2. ASP, *Fondo Comunale*, b. 588, c. 1259v.

CHAPTER III

CRISTOFANO AT WORK

It did not take long for Cristofano to show his qualities as an upright and energetic administrator. When he took up his job as Provveditore (11th Dec. 1630), there were '77 houses closed in Prato with 223 souls inside them',[1] and all these people quarantined at home were being kept at the town's expense. Cristofano notes in his *Libro* that

the Treasurer had (the allowances) paid to one who had the task of providing victuals for those shut up in their homes, but as errors had arisen, this task was given to the *Provveditore*, who, finding houses still closed after 22 or more days' quarantine, opened them insofar as he thought the situation warranted. And all these mouths were paid at the rate of one *giulio* a day.

The information given by Cristofano proves to be exact in every detail. From the letter of instruction sent by the Health Board in Florence to the officers in Prato on September 20th,

1. ASP, LS, c. 1-28. According to a letter of the *Podestà*'s dated December 14th, 1630, only 31 houses were closed in Prato (ASF, *Sanità*, Negozi b. 153, c. 731 and 744). The *Podestà* just states the total without giving any details. Instead, Cristofano lists the houses he opened from Dec. 11th, 1630 to Jan. 18th, 1631, specifying the date for each house and the number of persons quarantined in it. He states specifically (c. 3) that all these houses 'were closed before the election of the *Provveditore*'. His list totals 77 houses. As 13 houses were opened on his orders on Dec. 11th, by Dec. 14th when the *Podestà* wrote his letter there were still 64 houses closed in Prato. The information supplied by Cristofano is so detailed that it is difficult to doubt its general accuracy. Why the *Podestà* gives the total as 31, I cannot say.

1630 (after the first case of plague had been certified), we know that the officers had to give people under house-quarantine victuals worth one *giulio* per day;[1] this is confirmed in a letter of the Chancellor, Mainardi, dated October 22nd, 1630.[2] The minutes of the town council prove that from October 9th onwards a man had been hired to deliver the allowances to those confined in their homes.[3] The '*Istruzioni del Magistrato della Sanità di Firenze*' indicate that the quarantine had to last 22 days.[4]

Cristofano refers to 'errors' but he meant 'abuses'. From what he says and even more clearly from what he did, we gather that it suited some people to stay confined in their homes so as to get the daily allowance even after the quarantine period had expired. Point 5 of the list of tasks entrusted to the Provveditore's office[5] also suggests that, according to the Health officers, deaths in these houses were not always reported immediately, so that the town continued to pay for the 'ghosts' – the money being pocketed by the paying officer or the dead man's family or both.

The first thing Cristofano did as *Provveditore* was to have houses opened 'when they had done 22 or more days' quarantine in so far as he thought the situation warranted'. Obviously his idea was to cut out unjustified expenditure on the allowances. Cristofano was appointed *Provveditore* on 11th December. On the same day he had 13 houses opened with 35 persons inside them. Four days later, he opened another 9 houses containing 27 persons. Before the end of the month, he had opened 59 houses, and the remaining 18 were opened in the first 18 days of 1631.[6]

This was decisive action but Cristofano did not stop there.

1. See above p. 42.
2. ASF, *Sanità*, Negozi, b. 151, c. 1086.
3. See below, Appendix 1.
4. See below, Appendix 8.
5. See above, p. 64.
6. See Appendix 6.

As mentioned above, according to the instructions of the Board in Florence, Prato gave 1 *giulio* (i.e. 13⅓ *soldi*) per day to each person under house-quarantine. After Cristofano's appointment, this allowance was cut from 13⅓ *soldi* to 10 *soldi* because – as Cristofano asserts in his *Libro* – on 10 *soldi* a day, a person could 'easily sustain himself'.[1] And there were more changes to come. As the poorer confinees received a free bread ration, the allowance to them was cut from 10 to 5 *soldi* 'to relieve some part of the Community's heavy expenses'.[2] Another step was taken, too. As it was obviously an abuse that those who were not needy should get the allowance, it was decided that 'whosoever had means to sustain himself' should receive no allowance at all.[3]

Such decisions must have been taken by the whole assembly of the Health officers since this was the deliberative body – the *Provveditore* being only its executive arm. Yet the timing of the decisions and the circumstances in which they were made suggests they were instigated by Cristofano, who cherished nothing so dearly as the '*denaro del Pubblico*' and good administration. In all likelihood Cristofano was not very popular in those days, but the test of a good administrator is whether he has the strength of character and the honesty to put the interests of efficient administration before his own popularity.

While getting some of the houses opened, Cristofano also had to see about closing others but the list of houses closed during

---

1. Cristofano's information (ASP, LS, c. 3) is confirmed in the report that Chancellor Mainardi sent the Florence Health Board on 5th Feb. 1631 (ASF, *Sanità*, Negozi, b. 155, c. 261 and 280). The Chancellor wrote that the house confinees 'are each given 6 *crazie* per day'. As a *crazia* was equal to 20 *denari* (GALEOTTI, *Monete*, p. 274), six *crazie* were worth 120 *denari*, i.e., 10 *soldi*.

2. ASP, LS, c. 3.   3. ASP, LS, c. 19.

his time as *Provveditore*, does not begin before January 11th, 1631.[1] With the plague still reaping its fatal harvest, for one month from the day of his appointment, Cristofano continued to open houses but did not close a single one. Obviously he must have been more afraid of a deficit in the town's finances than he was of the plague itself. On January 11th 1631, however, he had 3 houses closed with 7 persons in them. The next day he closed another with 4 people in it, and the day after that another with 4 in it. Thus it went on. Between January 11th and October 24th he had closed 149 houses.

As mentioned above, Cristofano had ruled that 'whosoever had means to sustain himself' should not receive the allowance. For the rest, he distinguished between the infected and the contacts. If a man was infected but refused to go to the pest-house, then even though poor, he would be left without an allowance – since it was supposed 'that those who wanted to look after themselves at home could also sustain themselves without public moneys'.[2] It was a specious argument and Cristofano frankly confesses the real reason when he says: 'this was done to give the poor more heart to go to the lazaretto.'[3]

As shown in Appendix 3 (p. 147) those who died in the pest house of St Anne represent only 27 per cent of the total mortality. This proves how difficult Cristofano must have found it to send people to the pest house, partly because of their own reluctance, partly because of the conditions that existed there.

This brings us back to one of the thorniest problems, if not *the* thorniest problem that harassed Cristofano as *Provveditore* – the lazaretto.

It is reported that the Milan lazaretto held almost ten thousand 'patients' during the famine of 1629[4] and more than fifteen

1. ASP, LS, c. 19 ff.   2. ASP, LS, c. 19.
3. ASP, LS, c. 19.   4. TADINO, *Raguaglio*, p. 11.

thousand at the height of the plague in 1630.[1] At Bologna, during the 1630 plague, the pest-house of the Santissima Annunziata had reached a total of more than 500 patients and the pest-house of Santa Maria degli Angeli had more than 400.[2] At Florence the lazaretto at San Miniato held more than 900 patients.[3] In the summer of 1630, the pest-house of Verona housed over four thousand[4] and in August 1631 the pest-house of Padua had over two thousand.[5] At Turin in 1630-31, the lazaretto for contacts only, contained from 300 to 500 persons.[6] At Prato the pest-house in the convent of St Anne never held more than 60.

In the larger towns there was a tendency to put both the infected and the contacts into the pest-houses though in such cases the infected were generally kept apart from the contacts. The Milan pest-house had one department for the infected and another for the 'suspicious'. In other cities such as Turin, Rome and Palermo, there were separate pest-houses for the infected and the contacts. Prato had none of these arrangements; poverty precluded perfectionism. The rule was to put the contacts under house-quarantine and try to get the infected into the lazaretto.[7]

1. TADINO, *Raguaglio*, p. 117 and BOGNETTI, *Lazzaretto*, pp. 438-9.

2. BRIGHETTI, *Bologna*, pp. 179 ff.

3. ASF, *Sanità*, Negozi, b. 152, see reports of 28th-30th Nov. 163·0

4. PONA, *Il gran contagio*, p. 67.

5. FERRARI, *Lazzaretto di Padova*, p. 149; FERRARI, *Ufficio di Sanità*, p. 132.

6. ACT, *Ordinati*, vol. 180, c. 32v. (19th Dec. 1630) and 44 (18th Jan. 1631).

7. Cf. the first paragraphs in the list of tasks entrusted to the *Provveditore di Sanità* as specified when Cristofano was appointed (see above, p. 64). In his *Libro* (c. 32 v.), Cristofano writes that 'in houses where there have been sickness or deaths by contagion . . . at once the dead or the sick were brought away' and 'those who remained in the closed houses were sent a straw mattress straight away'. At c. 28v. as at c. 31, 58v., 64v. and else-

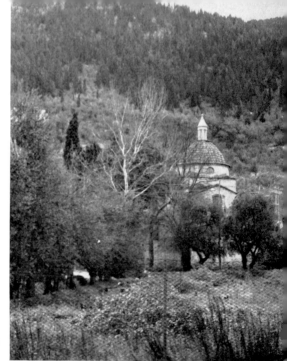

e convent of St Anne which was
nsformed into the lazaretto

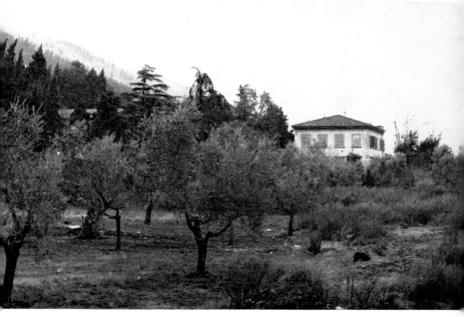

The *casa del poder murato* which housed the convalescents

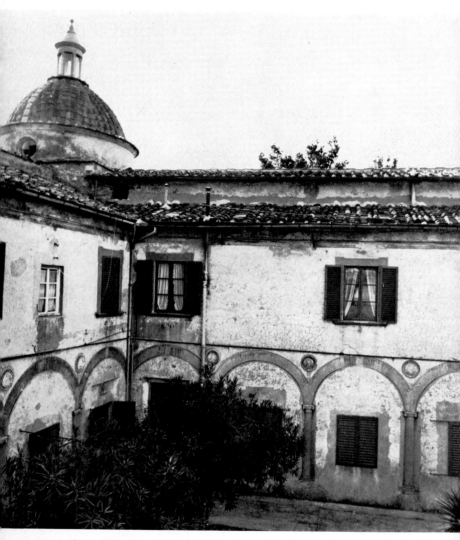

The inner courtyard of the Convent of St Anne as it appears to-day

After the pest-house had been transferred from the San Silvestro hospital to the Convent of St Anne as narrated above, Prato had at its disposal a convalescent-home as well as a pest-house. The patients who recovered and left the pest-house alive, 'were put into convalescence where they remained at least 22 days.'[1] However, as a precautionary measure they were not sent to the convalescent-home or released from it in dribs and drabs. They were organized into groups, and whatever the size of the group, when it arrived at the convalescent-home it took over the building entirely. When it was released from the home it was released as a whole. After this, 'the home was swept and cleaned and new convalescents were brought into it.'[2]

To sum up, Cristofano's standard procedure was this: (a) shut up all the contacts in their homes for 22 days' quarantine; (b) send the infected to the pest-house; (c) send the survivors to the convalescent-home; (d) keep the convalescents in the home for 22 days' quarantine. All this was simple in theory. In practice it was very tricky and full of complications. To understand why this was so, we must remember that Cristofano had to deal not only with the plague-germs but also with bureaucrats and financial problems, which were not lesser evils, and never are.

As we saw in the last chapter, it was Cristofano's job to manage the pest-house and the convalescent-home, where he

---

where when Cristofano refers to occupants of the pest-house he always calls them 'the sick', or 'the infirm'. And 'convalescents' is the term he always uses for those who leave the pest-house alive. This goes to show that only the infected were held in the Prato lazaretto.

See also RONDINELLI, *Contagio in Firenze*, p. 82 and the *Istruzioni* reproduced below in Appendix 8.

1. ASP, LS, c. 64v.   2. ASP, LS, c. 64v.

acted as representative of the Health officers of Prato. The Town Council paid the wages of those who worked in the pest-house but furniture, furnishings, implements and food were provided by the hospital *della Misericordia*. As this hospital was run by a Governor directly appointed by the Grand Duke of Florence, the arrangement was a natural source of bureaucratic conflict. The situation was aggravated by the fact that the governor, Captain Andrea Martinazzi, was an awkward customer; having been appointed by the Grand Duke he was deliberately contemptuous of the Prato Council and its representatives.[1] It is a sad commentary on human nature and social organization that even in the midst of sorrow and suffering when there were lives to be saved and pain to be alleviated, bureaucratic wrangling should have had so much effect on the efficiency of the hospital service. In fact, the hospital never provided adequate help for the pest-house. It sent furniture, furnishings and implements but not in adequate quantity. Even the supplies of food and medicines from the Hospital were never satisfactory. In his *Libro*, Cristofano never dwells on this point but every now and then we glimpse his continual frustration and disappointment. At c. 66v. he hints that 'we were hindered by much difficulty over the victuals'. Among the list of his expenses (c. 56 and 58) one finds the following entries:

6th March 1631 – for the convalescents who had risen up and come to the door (of the convalescent-home) because the hospital's superintendent refused to send food – 28 loaves of bread so that the convalescents might sustain themselves *lire* 2. 16. 0

13th March 1631 – firewood to burn the infected clothes of the convalescents, because the hospital's superintendent refused to provide it, oil and salt *lire* 4. 10. 0

1. ASP, *Diurno* 2, c. 175 (5th and 8th Dec. 1630).

24th March 1631 – one *barile* of oil and two *fiaschi* of vinegar because the hospital's superintendent provided only bread and wine   *lire* 1. 13. 0

5th May 1631 – bread for the convalescents who had not had their meal because the hospital's superintendent did not send the pro-visions   *lire* 2. 17. 0

In addition to food and firewood, Cristofano had to buy pots, pans, implements and medicines which were badly needed both in the pest-house and in the convalescent-home.

He drew on a fund he himself had set up to supply the pest-house with things the Hospital omitted to send. Unfortunately, Cristofano's funds were limited and he could not make up for all the hospital's shortcomings so that, as he writes, 'the sick and the convalescents lacked many necessary things.'[1]

I have checked the accounts of the Hospital and found that for the period 1st July 1630 to 30th June 1631, its receipts totalled 7,475 ducats while its payments – including supplies to the lazaretto – came to 5,305. At the height of the epidemic, therefore, while failing to supply enough food, medicines blankets and firewood to the pest-house, the Hospital had a surplus to the tune of 2,170 ducats.[2] It is to Cristofano's credit that in his *Libro*, the hints at this unpleasant state of affairs are always restrained. He never lets himself go in a personal out-burst or an attack on Captain Martinazzi. Besides being a parsimonious administrator Cristofano was also a prudent man with a good deal of self-control. On February 25th, 1631, the Health Board in Florence was informed that the Hospital governor was making difficulties about supplying the food to the pest-house. The letter was obviously inspired by Cristofano

1. ASP, LS, c. 64v.
2. ASP, *Fondo Comunale*, b. 587, c. 1362.

but it was written and signed by the *Podestà*.[1] On June 2nd, 1631 another letter was addressed to the Health Board in Florence. The letter explained that the epidemic was ravaging the countryside and the officers wanted to comply with the order of the Board and admit the infected from the villages to the pest-house of St Anne. However – so the letter goes on – the governor of the Hospital 'who until now has provided the food to the lazaretto though in inadequate quantity, does not intend to feed those who will be sent to the pest-house from the countryside'. The handwriting is that of Cristofano but the letter is signed 'The Health officers of Prato'.[2]

The reaction of the Board in Florence to the letter of June 2nd was prompt and firm: on June 5th the Board wrote that Captain Martinazzi had to be reminded that during an epidemic it is the task of an Hospital administration to 'tend and succour the poor even if it means some inconvenience'; the task is not 'to try to increase the receipts of suchlike pious place.'[3] The relations between the Pratesi and Captain Martinazzi remained very strained and early in 1632 the Town Council of Prato openly declared that the Captain 'does not govern the Hospital well'.[4]

As a result of conflicts over bureaucratic responsibility and probably of clashes of personalities, the situation in the lazaretto continued to be as bad as ever, with Cristofano resorting to expedients month after month. At last, in June 1631, 'as the sick and the convalescents lacked many necessities,' a group of religious laymen, the '*Veneranda Compagnia del Pellegrino*', asked the Health officers of Prato for authorization to take upon themselves the administration and provisioning of the

1. ASF, *Sanità*, Negozi, b. 155, c. 813 and 820.
2. ASF, *Sanità*, Negozi, b. 158, c. 34.
3. ASF, *Sanità*, Copialettere, b. 57, c. 165.
4. ASP, *Diurno* 3, c. 115v. (2nd Feb. 1632).

lazaretto and the convalescent-home as an act of charity. The officers agreed since it was the only way to ensure that 'the sick and convalescents might have sufficient victuals, fire and medicines'. The decision was taken on June 15th, 1631[1] and on June 17th the pest-house and the home passed under the administration of the *Veneranda Compagnia*.[2] For Cristofano this meant the end of a source of continual worry and for the patients it meant the end of inadequate treatment. But meanwhile months had passed and the epidemic was on the wane.

However, Captain Martinazzi was not Cristofano's only problem. There was also the large deficit in the town's finances, which regularly prevented him from doing what he should have done. To discharge people who had recovered in the pest-house and finished their quarantine in the convalescent-home, the rule was as follows: 'make them wash thoroughly, burn all the clothes they have on their backs and dress them in new garments from head to foot and give them 10 *soldi* for alms...'[3] So much for the rule. In practice the money, to buy new clothes for the outgoing convalescents, was often not available. On February 25th, 1631, the *Podestà* wrote to Florence that there were '44 sick in the lazaretto and 5 convalescents in the home whereof 35 are well enough to be dismissed' but they were not being 'dismissed' because there was no money to provide them with new clothes after burning their old ones. 'We have witnessed' – the *Podestà* goes on – 'that to discharge the patients from the lazaretto and send them back to their homes with the garments they have worn in their sickness has caused not only a relapsing of those discharged but also the infection

1. ASP, *Diurno* 3, c. 33.   2. ASP, LS, c. 64v.   3. ASP, LS, c. 55v.

of others in the house'.[1] The Chancellor, V. Mainardi, too, in his letter dated February 5th, 1631, mentions 'the evil effect that stems from not having purged the houses and the people by burning the beds and the garments of the infected' because of lack of funds.[2]

When Cristofano writes in his *Libro* that the allowance was not to be given to infected persons who wanted to stay in their homes in order 'to give the poor more heart to go to the lazaretto', he shows he had grasped a central idea of his time, i.e. whereas one might allow the well-off victims to stay in their homes, it was essential to send the poor ones to the lazaretto. This was quite clear to Cristofano, but it was easier said than done. With the difficulties caused by Captain Martinazzi, the capacity of the pest-house at the Convent of St Anne had been reduced; it could not possibly house all those who should have been sent there. As if this was not enough, with no funds to buy new clothes, Cristofano could not even get those who had recovered out of the pest-house. He was between the devil and the deep blue sea. All he could do was to manage somehow by breaking the health regulations. On two occasions when the numbers in the pest-house reached 58 (31st Jan. 1631) and 55 (11th March 1631), Cristofano sent 15 off to the convalescent-home the first time and 11 the second time.[3] In both cases one has the impression that Cristofano did not really have inmates ready for convalescence but that he had to clear them out of the lazaretto, whose maximum capacity must have been about forty. The letters quoted above from the *Podestà* and the Chancellor make it clear also that Cristofano

1. ASF, *Sanità*, Negozi, b. 155, c. 813 and 820.
2. ASF, *Sanità*, Negozi, b. 155, c. 261 and 280.
3. See below, Appendix 3.

broke the rules and released convalescents who were allowed to go home in the clothes they had worn in the lazaretto. An examination of the statistics given by Cristofano for the convalescent-home also shows that the convalescents rarely spent all the regulation 22 days' quarantine there. Maybe in some cases, as Cristofano asserts at c. 64v. of his *Libro*, the quarantine period was reduced because the patients had 'been healthy a sufficient number of days in the pest-house', i.e. had done part of the quarantine there. But at c. 66v., when mentioning the problems that led to the lazaretto's administration being handed over to the *Compagnia del Pellegrino*, Cristofano himself admits that some convalescents had been released 'before time' because 'we had been hindered by much difficulty over the victuals'.

Cristofano could hardly have liked breaking the health regulations. This is clear from the fact that as the epidemic waned and the average daily number of inmates in the lazaretto fell off, he sent a larger and larger proportion of the sick to the lazaretto.[1] Yet the fact remains that the narrow-mindedness of bureaucrats and the financial difficulties forced him to break

---

1. A comparison between the two following sets of figures is revealing:

period	average number of patients in the pest-house	deaths in the pest-house as per cent of total number of deaths in town
January 14th-31st	49	10
February 1st-28th	47	26
March 1st-31st	42	35
April 1st-30th	24	35
May 1st-31st	20	33

The basic data on which the above figures are calculated can be found in the Appendices.

the health regulations at the very moment when the plague was at its worst – and this must have cost him suffering and continual fits of rage.

Chronically short of funds, confronted daily with urgent and tragic needs, Cristofano had to resort constantly to all kinds of expedients. As early as December 1630, at the time of his appointment as *Provveditore*, it was obvious that the available funds would not be enough, above all for the extra expenses that were bound to arise. The transfer of the pest-house was being planned. Rooms for the new pest-house and the convalescent-home had been found at St Anne's but they were not equipped, i.e. they did not have the necessary beds, blankets, sheets, or firewood. It was winter, which meant more of these things were needed – and the hospital *della Misericordia* was proving anything but generous. Cristofano turned to public charity. It was the only chance. Within a week of his appointment, he organized a 'search for things and money'. To add weight to this initiative, to get people to donate, and to speed up the operation, he himself took part in it. With two deputies, he went from house to house begging and explaining to the citizens why it was so important to set up the pest-house outside the town as soon as possible:

Two deputies together with the *Provveditore* have gone on this search for things and moneys so as to make greater speed in the business since it is to the great detriment of the country that the lazaretto should be within the city-walls.[1]

Between December 18th, 1630, and January 28th, 1631, Cristofano collected by begging:[2]

1. ASP, LS, c. 28v.   2. ASP, LS, cc. 28 v.-30v.

old feather-mattresses	1
bed-cloths	3
feather-pillows	3
blankets	4
woollen mattresses	1
tow mattresses	8
large sheets	1
sheets	22
new palliasses	11
old palliasses	2
wooden bedframes	3

Many of these things were second-hand but as far as infection was concerned they were considered clean. Cristofano therefore decided to keep them all for the convalescent-home and for the use of the surgeon in the pest-house. He gave the surgeon one tow mattress, one wooden bedframe, one feather-pillow, one feather-mattress, one pair of sheets as well as a couple of palliasses that he had bought from funds we shall mention later. He sent the rest of the things collected to the convalescent-home. Thus, the convalescent-home problem was partially solved but the more serious problem of the pest-house remained. Cristofano had to find some other expedient for this.

In 1576 the plague was raging in Sicily and the physician Giovan Filippo Ingrassia published his 'Information on the pestiferous and contagious sickness which is afflicting and has afflicted this city of Palermo and other cities and areas of this Kingdom'. As a motto for his work he chose: 'Gold, fire, the gallows'. '*Ignis, furca, aurum sunt medicina mali*' – gold for the expense, the gallows to punish those who violate the health regulations and to frighten the others, and fire to eliminate infected things. In the towns stricken by plague, next to the gallows, sinister bonfires of infected goods were always burning.

Everything a plague-victim had touched was considered infected and capable of transmitting the disease. But the potential of each object as a transmitter varied greatly. It was thought that the contagious disease or 'sticking' disease as some called it, could 'stick' more easily to certain materials such as feathers, furs, wool, blankets, rags, etc. In the same way, it was believed the disease would 'stick' more readily to the hairy parts of the human body than to the smooth ones. The idea of how this actually happened was as vague as it was ingenuous. But it was not absurd. We know now that bubonic plague is transmitted by fleas[1]; materials such as cloth, fur, feathers, carpets, etc., just like the hairy parts of the human body, generally offer easier shelter for the fleas. Behind the over-simple and ingenuously mistaken theorizing of the time there was an intelligent and accurate observation of the facts.

There were two possible treatments foreseen for infected goods – disinfecting or destruction by fire. A basic general principle was that goods which were most likely to act as carriers of the disease (e.g. beds, pillows, blankets, clothes, cloths, etc.) should be burnt if they had been declared infected. Other goods should be disinfected. But even the more severe and intransigent of the doctors and health officers never gave their full support to this principle.

1. It seems that the chief agent in the propagation of plague is the rat flea (*Xenophilla Cheopis*). There is evidence however that the human flea (*Pulex irritans*) may occasionally spread plague from man to man, especially when the human flea is superabundant, as was certainly the case in Medieval and Renaissance times. According to most epidemiologists, only great numbers can compensate for the intrinsic inferiority of *Pulex irritans* as a vector of plague. See Hirst, *Conquest of Plague*, pp. 236-46.

Consciously or unconsciously, the principle was modified by factors that were essentially economic. Pre-industrial societies were basically poor and they could not afford a destruction of goods *en masse* in obedience to vague and abstruse concepts of health and hygiene. In general it was held that if the goods supposedly infected were new or valuable they should be saved, i.e. disinfected, whereas if they were old or of little value they should be burnt. Obviously position and influence came into play here. Nobles, rich men, and merchants could and did manage to save their possessions from the flames. The poor had no power to do so. Moreover there was also an economic factor which, even if it was not expressed must have been felt instinctively: disinfection cost money and while it may have been worth paying this cost for goods of some value, it was illogical to do so for what was comparatively worthless.

Such problems presented themselves to Cristofano in Prato as they did to any other health officer in any other town. But for Cristofano they were further complicated by the urgent needs of the pest-house. How could he possibly burn infected mattresses and blankets when in the pest-house there were sick people lying on the damp floor with nothing to protect them from cold and humidity? He requisitioned all the goods and chattels in the houses 'where there have been sick or dead'[1] and sorted the good from the bad. The criteria for this division must have been purely subjective, 'good' meaning what was well preserved or valuable and 'bad' whatever was old or of little value. 'The bad stuff' was set on fire in the gravel-bed of

1. The owners of the goods requisitioned were reimbursed at the town's expense. In Prato the rule was to reimburse the owners fifty per cent of the 'just' value of what was requisitioned. To those whose bed was burned the community passed a new mattress which was valued at 9 *lire*. This amount was deducted from the reimbursement. For all this see ASP, LS, c. 32v.

the Bisenzio. These ominous bonfires burning on the gravel of the river-bed destroyed:[1]

blankets	21
feather-mattresses	54
palliasses	114
mattresses	46
feather-pillows	50
garments	13
hats	2
bedspreads	3

The household effects that were infected but considered 'good', were disinfected and then sent to the pest-house, which had a crying need for them: 'as they are good they have been sent to the lazaretto to serve for the sick so that they may rest with greater comfort'.[2] This was anything but orthodox practice. For the umpteenth time economic pressures had compelled Cristofano to make decisions that, from the medical point of view, were very questionable.[3]

From the first day he took office as *Provveditore*, lack of funds was Cristofano's chief problem. As I have already mentioned, within a week of his appointment he organized 'a search for things and moneys' appealing to public charity. A section of the *Libro della Sanità* is devoted to the 'moneys accepted for the love of God from divers persons for the succour of the

1. ASP, LS, c. 87, '*Intavolatura di tutte le robe che si sono abbruciate nel tempo della peste.*'

2. ASP, LS, c. 32 v.

3. Cristofano was neither the first nor the last health officer to resort to the dangerous expedient described above in the text. In 1633 the superintendent of the pest-house of Florence resorted to the same expedient in order to have an adequate supply of blankets and mattresses (RONDINELLI, *Relazione*, p. 182).

poor sick and convalescents who lack many necessities, and handed to Cristofano Ceffini *Provveditore* of the Health Board this day 18th December 1630'.[1] In all there were forty donations distributed as follows:[2]

lire	soldi	denari	number of the donations
—	6	8	1
—	10	—	2
—	13	4	1
1	—	—	2
2	—	—	13
2	3	4	1
2	6	8	2
2	13	4	1
3	—	—	2
4	—	—	6
6	—	—	1
7	—	—	4
14	—	—	3
21	—	—	1

The total was 166 *lire* and 10 *soldi*. The most generous of the donors, who gave 21 *lire*, was a certain Francesco di Domenico Bizzocchi. The Carthusian Fathers were among those who gave 14 *lire*. A third of the donors gave two *lire* and less than a tenth of them gave more than four *lire*. All together, they were modest sums. As we have seen, ten *soldi* was the figure Cristofano estimated as sufficient to buy one person food for one day – and Cristofano was not the man to exaggerate in such appraisals. Thus two *lire* would roughly represent the cost of a day's food for an average family of four. It should be remembered that the 'search' was not only for 'moneys' but also for

1. ASP, LS, c. 31.   2. ASP, LS, cc. 31-32.

'things' and that a plague-stricken town was also a poverty-stricken one. The fact remains, however, that the people of Prato did not shine for their prodigality.

Cristofano rounded off the small fund he had collected by adding the proceeds of a fine to it. Two men, Sabatino da Colonica and Simone da Fossi had been caught entering Prato without their health passes. For this infringement of the regulations, they were sentenced to be hung by the wrists with a weight slung round their ankles, which was the usual punishment. But as money was needed and the two had offered to pay, a 70 *lire* fine was substituted for this vertical form of torture by racking. This sum alone was little less than half the total collected in the 'search' which means not that the fine was heavy but that the collection was low.

Cristofano used his small fund to cover extra expenses. The largest of these was the 'alms' given to convalescents who had completed their quarantine whereupon they were released and sent to their homes. Under this 'alms' heading, from December 12th, 1630 to July 29th, 1631, Cristofano spent 110 *lire*, 3 *soldi* and 4 *denari*, i.e. a little less than half the money collected. Most of the remainder of the fund was spent on goods that the pest-house needed and the hospital did not want to provide, namely 'pots, basins, and sponges to wash the convalescents with' (16th December 1630), two palliasses for the bed of the surgeon in the pest-house (27th Feb. 1631), oil, incense and candles 'given to the surgeon for the needs of the pest-house' (22nd March 1631), etc., etc.[1]

Whatever aspect one considers of Cristofano's activity as Health *Provveditore*, one leitmotiv is always there – the funds at his disposal were never enough. The fund for extra expenses, a combination of 'search' donations and fines, totalled 236 *lire* and 10 *soldi*. Cristofano drew on the fund to pay expenses with

1. ASP, LS, cc. 55v.-58.

his characteristic caution and thriftiness. But by July 29th, 1631, he had spent 249 *lire*, 12 *soldi*, and 8 *denari*, i.e. exactly 13 *lire*, 2 *soldi*, 8 *denari*, more than he had had in the fund. Cristofano made up the difference out of his own pocket. Not as a donation, however. In the accounts the sum is credited to him. At that time it was not unusual for an eminent person in office to advance funds to his own office. We must recognize that Cristofano stuck to the rules of *noblesse oblige*. The sum he advanced, though not really very substantial was still much larger than most of his fellow citizens had donated during the 'search'. Yet it must be mentioned that on that occasion one looks in vain for Cristofano's name among the donors.

CHAPTER IV

THE COURSE OF MORTALITY

For mortality in Prato during the epidemic we possess three major sources: (a) the *Books of the Deceased* of the town; (b) the daily number of deceased as given by Cristofano in his book covering the period from October 1st, 1630 to November 30th, 1631; (c) the daily number of deceased as given by the Podestà Giulio Morelli in his letters to the Health Board in Florence covering the period from November 21st to December 31st 1630.

The Books of the Deceased of the town are lists of names arranged alphabetically. They were compiled by officials on the basis of reports by the parish parsons but they are totally unreliable, especially in time of epidemics when under-registration was very common.[1] As I have already mentioned

1. A check I made for July to December gave the following results:

number of deceased in July	31
August	32
Sept.	35
Oct.	22
Nov.	180
Dec.	163

The under-registration is especially obvious for the month of October which was one of the worst periods of the epidemic. No deaths are registered in the Books from October 10th to October 27th.

On the other hand, the number of deaths registered for the months of July and August is definitely high for a town of about 6,000 people.

there is some disagreement between Cristofano's figures and those of the *Podestà* but they closely agree as to the trend prevailing from mid-November to the end of December.

During the month of August the plague was recognized in Florence and also in the small village of Tavola, in the territory of Prato. As I mentioned above, possibly the infection had made an inroad into Prato by August although officially the first case of plague was recognized on September 19th.[1]

In September however the epidemic developed rapidly and probably October was the worst month. The weather in that first part of the Autumn was unusually warm,[2] and if it favoured the survival and proliferation of the fleas it may have also favoured the diffusion of the epidemic.

With the cold weather typically the epidemic began to weaken its grip.[3] According to the information supplied by

1. See above, pp. 41-2.
2. ASF, *Sanità*, Negozi, b. 151, c. 407 (9th October 1630).
3. Available evidence seems to indicate that the season of the year has a very powerful influence on the prevalence of plague and the duration of the epidemic. Why plague is so strongly controlled by seasonal influences is one of the many problems to be solved. Season, with its meteorological factors, is a composite force and as such operates in more than one way on the agents and media connected with plague. For instance it affects a man's constitution and powers of resistance to infectious diseases in various ways through its influence on the air, soil and food which react on man; it affects the plague bacillus as regards reproduction and virulence; it affects animal and insect life as well. The difficulty lies in differentiating among the main factors.

The range of temperature favourable to plague varies considerably in different localities, the most favourable being between 56° F and 75° F. Mean temperatures above 83° F and below 50° F are as a rule unsuitable for epidemic prevalence. The varying hygrometric condition of the soil and its fluctuating temperature are likely to affect the multiplication and possible virulence of the plague bacillus. They are even more likely to exercise a great influence on the life of insects which may carry infection to and from animals susceptible to plague, such as rats. That a mean temperature of 83° F

the *Podestà* and by Cristofano, the number of deaths declined slowly from the end of November and more markedly during December. This is confirmed by other facts. On December 31st, 1630, the officers met with the *Podestà* and as public health was improving while finance was deteriorating, they decided to reduce the salaries of some people in the Public Health service.[1] The same day the *Podestà* wrote to the Board in Florence mentioning the advisability of lifting the ban that forbade all communications and trade between Prato and Florence, although he admitted that a number of people in Prato did not share his views.[2]

Early in January the Health Board in Florence decreed the 'general quarantine' for all communities in the Florentine territory. This quarantine was to last for 40 days starting from January 10th.[3] The 'general quarantine' was a measure that authorities usually adopted during an epidemic to finish it off

_____

should exert a marked control over an epidemic of plague while the bacillus flourishes in man at 98° F and in birds at 107° F leads one to suppose that the influence is not a direct one on the *pasteurella pestis* itself. This view seems particularly valid when one considers how much the infection is a house infection where direct sunshine plays a very unimportant part, the microbe never being exposed to any high aerial temperature or to any exceptional low temperature which might destroy it. Winter may favour the development of pneumonic complications but if this does not happen, the severe cold of the winter generally has a deterring effect on bubonic plague. The figures given by Ceffini and by the *Podestà* show that the epidemic was dying down rapidly during December. The figures given by Ceffini indicate that the downward trend continued until March. With the spring any further improvement stopped and in June, with the humidity and the heat of the early summer the plague actually had a revival.

1. ASP, *Diurno* 2, c. 182v. and below Appendix 1.
2. ASF, *Sanità*, Negozi, b. 153, c. 1358.
3. ASF, *Sanità*, Bandi, vol. 2, c. 86.

more quickly. It consisted in limiting the movements of all people and especially in forbidding assembly.[1] The ordinance was sent to Prato on January 5th and it was publicly proclaimed 'in the usual places with a trumpet call' on January 9th and again on January 13th.[2]

The advisability of a general quarantine is open to question and it was in fact hotly debated.[3] There is no doubt that if accompanied by immediate isolation of all contacts and infected people, the idea of forbidding assemblies and severely limiting the movements and intercourse of people is a perfectly sound one. But when the source of infection is still active in their homes, a general quarantine just increased the chances

1. Point 1 of the ordinance forbade people to come to Florence with the exception of one person for every household who had to have a regular health pass. Point 2 forbade people to visit one another in their homes 'especially to have meetings, games, dances or entertainments'. It was not prohibited 'to go to church, to the mill, to the markets, to the baker's, to the butcher's and to other shops, provided that it is only out of necessity'. Point 5 forbade also to the noblemen and citizens of Florence who lived in their villas in the *contado* to have games, feasts or meetings during the period of the quarantine. Neither were they allowed to visit one another in their villas.

2. ASF, *Sanità*, Negozi, b. 154, c. 602 (14th Jan. 1631).

3. For Milan see TADINO, *Raguaglio*, p. 127. The Milanese physician was especially opposed to having a general quarantine in the summer months. In Busto Arsizio during the plague of 1630 the 'general quarantine' was declared on April 18th. According to a witness 'no sooner had four days passed from its beginning than where before seven or eight had been dying per day, the number was doubled to fifteen or sixteen per day; and in the space of eight days many houses found they were infected, those of the rich as much as those of the poor, so that almost two parts out of three were infected' (JOHNSSON, *Busto Arsizio*, pp. 20-21). In Florence the general quarantine was opposed by some people (RONDINELLI, *Contagio di Firenze*, pp. 60 ff. and CATELLACCI, *Ricordi*, p. 387). In Bologna the general quarantine was proclaimed in September 1630; on the discussions about its advisability cf. BRIGHETTI, *Bologna*, pp. 62 ff.

of infection for the people. If one looks at the figures given by Cristofano, one notices that during January and February mortality kept falling but at a lower rate. Probably this was due to the normal course of the epidemic; but it would be difficult to maintain that the general quarantine had any positive results.

At any rate, although at a lower rate, the downward trend of mortality continued. On February 25th the *Podestà* wrote to Florence that 'thank God, things pertaining to public health are going very well',[1] and according to Cristofano the number of deaths was down to 15 per week against 94 in the last two weeks of October.[2] On March 10th the *Podestà* wrote again to Florence that in Prato things were going well. The Board had instructed him to forbid the traditional Lent sermons in the churches and he reported that he had already taken this precaution.[3] On March 18th the *Podestà* wrote that 'the disease has so diminished since mid-February that we can hope to be completely free from it soon.'[4] In fact, according to Cristofano's figures, the week from March 11th to March 17th saw the lowest level of mortality in Prato since the outbreak of the epidemic.

The optimism of the *Podestà* however was ill founded. After about the middle of March, with the coming of spring, the disease picked up strength and although at a very low level of intensity it kept creeping into the town, with the weekly number of deaths fluctuating around seven. The *Podestà* kept sending reassuring letters to Florence petitioning the lifting of

1. ASF, *Sanità*, Negozi, b. 155, c. 813 and 820.
2. Excluding four who died in the pest-house at the Convent of St Anne.
3. ASF, *Sanità*, Negozi, b. 155, c. 1194 (10th March 1631). In 1631 Easter fell on April 20th.
4. ASF, *Sanità*, Negozi, b. 155, c. 1402.

the ban,[1] but the Board in Florence hesitated. Prato was not completely free of plague. Moreover, the Board had information that although in Prato itself the plague had dropped drastically since late February, it was now flaring up in the neighbouring countryside.[2] In the first part of April the Board sent one of its physicians, Dr Giuseppe Morvidi, to Prato to appraise the situation.[3] The report by Morvidi must have been unfavourable as the ban was not lifted. This was wise because in June the epidemic had its last spasm. Then, on July 11th the Town Council noted that 'for twenty two days there have not been cases of infection nor deaths from contagion' and consequently it decided to reopen the schools and to request again from Florence the lifting of the ban.[4] Two days later the *Podestà* wrote to Florence accordingly.[5] In all likelihood the Town Council, as well as the *Podestà* deliberately ignored a few cases of 'suspicious deaths' that occurred in Prato between June 19th and July 13th.[6] Again the Board sent Dr Morvidi to Prato. Although the epidemic was obviously over, endemically the plague was always present and sporadic cases of suspected infection appeared from time to time.[7] Now, however, the report by Dr Morvidi was favourable. Possibly the Commissioner agreed with the officers that a few doubtful cases were not enough to justify the continuous isolation of the whole city. On July 17th the Board lifted the ban: the people

1, ASF, *Sanità*, Negozi, b. 155, c. 1465 (20th March 1630).

2. ASF, *Sanità*, Copialettere, b. 57, c. 79 (24th April 1631), c. 89 (30th April 1631), b. 58, c. 90v. (11th July 1631), c. 99 (15th July 1631); *Sanità*, Negozi, b. 158, c. 34 (2nd June 1631).

3. ASF, *Sanità*, Copialettere, b. 57, c. 59v. (9th April 1631).

4. ASP, *Diurno* 3, c. 45.

5. ASF, *Sanità*, Negozi, b. 157, c. 475 (13th July 1631).

6. According to Cristofano nine deaths occurred in Prato from June 19th to July 13th. On the conflicting evidence see above p. 71.

7. See preceding footnote.

and the products of Prato were admitted to Florence providing they were accompanied by health passes.[1]

In the countryside the epidemic was still rampant and caused no little worry to the Health officers. One fact impressed them especially. Diacinto Gramigna the surgeon had served in the pest-house at the Convent of St Anne from February 16th, 1631. Although in daily and close contact with the infected he never contracted the plague, but soon after the infected from the countryside were admitted to the pest-house, Gramigna fell sick and developed the typical pestiferous bubo.[2] This fact may be of some interest also to modern epidemiologists. To the Health officers of the time, it simply meant that the plague of the countryside was more contagious and pestiferous than the plague which had ravaged the town and this was not a reassuring thought. However Gramigna managed to recover and by August the epidemic was finally dying out in the *contado* too. On September 21st, 1631 the *Veneranda Compagnia del Pellegrino* 'returned the lazaretto to the officers as there were no more sick there'.[3] To celebrate the event, a Dominican friar, father Campana 'gave a notable sermon in the cathedral' and in the evening 'festivities were held with fireworks and bells'.[4]

According to Cristofano the number of deaths in Prato was:[5]

October 1630	368
November	317
December	213
January 1631	110
February	66

1. ASF, *Sanità*, Copialettere, b. 58, c. 107,
2. ASF, *Sanità*, Negozi, b. 159, c. 349 (9th July 1631).
3. ASP, LS, c. 64v.   4. ASP, *Diurno* 3, c. 64 (21st Sept. 1631).
5. See Appendix 7.

March	30
April	37
May	35
June	37
July	5
August	4
September	3
October	6
November	5

In the figures given by Cristofano, those who died in the pest-house at the Convent of St Anne outside the walls were not included. They amounted to 100 people between January 14th and June 16th. Until June 2nd the sick from the country-side were not admitted to the lazaretto which was reserved for the infected from the town.[1] We can therefore safely add about one hundred units to the 1,213 deaths from October 1630 to June 1631. There is no information about the number of deaths in September 1630, but one may suggest that between September 1st, 1630 and the end of June 1631, about 1,500 people died in Prato. I have already indicated above that the figures reported by Cristofano refer to 'deaths from contagion' with the inclusion of the 'doubtful cases'.[2] If before the epidemic Prato numbered about 6,000 souls within the walls, the epidemics wiped out about 25 per cent of the population. According to father Campana, who delivered the sermon in the *Duomo* when the pest-house was closed, the Pratesi had to be thankful to God because 'in Prato the disease had not been as awful and severe as in other places'.[3] Mortality

1. ASF, *Sanità*, Negozi, b. 158, c. 34 (2nd June 1631).

2. See above p. 70. In view of the fact that the ban was lifted by the Board in Florence on August 17th, all deaths recorded by Cristofano for the period August to November must be regarded as 'doubtful cases'.

3. ASP, *Diurno* 3, c. 64 (21st Sept. 1631).

had been higher in other places, especially in those which were hit by the plague during the summer. Possibly Prato suffered less because the plague reached it when the fleas were less active, sexually and otherwise. But this father Campana could not know. Anyhow it is a significant commentary on the tragedy the plague represented that people felt they had to be grateful when it had taken no more than a few months to kill off some twenty-five per cent of the population.

Mortality rates give the proportion of deaths to total population. Fatality rates relate those who die to the infected. We have no data to estimate the fatality rates for the town of Prato, during the epidemic, but the statistics on the pest-house provide some food for thought. Having no list of names, the best way to use the figures on the pest-house is to calculate the ratio of those who died either over those who entered the establishment or over those who left it whether dead or alive.[1]

1. The two methods would be practically the same if the statistics covered the whole period in which the pest-house operated. But as explained in the previous chapters, the pest-house of Prato was handed over to the *Compagnia del Pellegrino* on June 17th. On that date Cristofano interrupted his statistics. There were 30 patients in the house which means that the number of those who entered the establishment from January 14th to June 16th is greater than the number of those who left it during the same period. We have no idea of what happened to those 30 patients.

If one calculates the ratio of those who died over those who left the pest-house whether dead or alive, one has to take into account that those who left alive were taken out in groups, while the deceased left the establishment day by day. On May 30th, 1631, a group of 10 convalescents were discharged. The statistics of Cristofano continue until June 16th, but the deaths during the period May 31st – June 16th cannot be taken into account because the corresponding number of survivals would have appeared at some date after June 16th when the next group of convalescents was discharged. In

The result is practically the same[1] i.e. only half of those who were hospitalized in the lazaretto lost their lives. The rate is definitely low not only in the light of the appalling sanitary conditions of a pest-house of the seventeenth century but also in the light of our current scientific knowledge of plague. One would be inclined to dismiss the figures of Prato if similar data available for other pest-houses did not yield the same results. Rates of 50 to 60 per cent prevailed in 1630 also in the pest-houses of San Miniato and San Francesco in Florence, in the pest-house of Empoli (Tuscany), in that of Trento (Trentino) and in that of Carmagnola (Piedmont).[2]

It might be supposed that some of those confined to the pest-house were not infected with plague. There is evidence for Bologna and for Florence that some unfortunate people who fell sick for one reason or the other, especially if poor, were sent to the pest-houses without actually carrying *pasteurella pestis*.[3]

---

calculating the proportion of the deceased over the total number of those who left the pest-house I therefore limited the observation to the period January 14th to May 30th.

If one calculates the ratio of those who died over those who entered the establishment one has to take into consideration the fact that in general people infected with plague die within a period of two to six days. Calculating the proportion of those who died over those who entered the pest-house I therefore referred the number of those who died from January 14th to June 16th to those who entered the pest-house from January 14th to June 10th.

1. Those who died over the period January 14th to May 30th were 82 and those who left it alive were 72. Total number of discharged 154. Proportion of deceased: 53 per cent.

Those who died from January 14th to June 16th were 100. Those who entered the establishment from January 14th to June 10th were 193. Proportion of deaths over admissions: 52 per cent.

2. For all this see my essay on *Plague in Empoli*, to be published.

3. See preceding foot-note.

If this happened in Florence and Bologna there is no reason why it should not have happened also in Prato. However, once in the pest-house the risk of catching the disease was obviously high. Probably the death rate in the pest house was comparatively low because a considerable number of those infected had died before they could be sent to hospital. Consequently those actually admitted constitute an already selected group.

Our scientific knowledge about plague is essentially derived from the plague epidemics that developed in India and in Manchuria in the nineteenth and early 20th centuries. It was observed that in untreated patients suffering from the usual type of bubonic plague leading to bacteraemia the average fatality rate amounted from 60 to 90 per cent. Though it may have taken place sooner or later, death during the acute stage of bubonic plague usually occurred within a period of 3 to 5 days from the onset of the illness, so that patients who survived for longer than five days had considerably increased chances of recovery.[1] Pneumonic plague is a more fatal disease. According to the Indian and Manchurian experience unless adequate specific and modern treatment is administered, patients suffering from primary pneumonic plague almost invariably die within a few days, sometimes even within less than a day. No authentic case of pulmonary plague has been known to survive before the discovery and application of antibiotics. According to Dr Choksy[2] who analysed 9,500 cases in Bombay fatality rates were for

simple bubonic plague	77%
septicaemic plague	90%
pneumonic plague	97%

1. POLLITZER, *Plague*, p. 418; WU, *Manchurian Plague*, p. 82.
2. Quoted by SIMPSON, *Treatise*, p. 313.

In the light of these modern experiences, the fatality rate observed in the pest-house of Prato was obviously that of the simple bubonic plague.

The plague did not affect the population of Prato in an egalitarian way. If we limit our attention to the little army which fought against the plague, we find that the high ranks were hardly touched. None of the Health officers died. The man in charge of the health passes, under-chancellor Novellucci, who belonged to one of the wealthiest families in town[1] survived the epidemic and died in 1648.[2] The physicians too happily survived the epidemics. The two community physicians, Lattanzio Magiotti and Giobatta Serrati were alive at the end of September 1631, when in a petition to the Town Council they exalted their own activities during the plague.[3] As to the other three physicians, according to the city's books of the deceased, Pier Francesco Fabbruzzi died in 1635, Giuliano Losti in 1648 and Jacopo Lionetti in 1638. In grim contrast the lower ranks paid a high toll to the plague. One of the surgeons succumbed;[4] the gravediggers and the attendants in the pest-house died like flies.[5] The differential mortality that we can document within the group of the Public Health force is reported macroscopically for the whole town. Writing to the Health Board in Florence on November 25th, 1630, the *Podestà* of Prato re-

1. FIUMI, *Prato*, p. 441.   2. ASP, *Fondo Comunale*, b. 3081.
3. ASP, *Diurno* 3, c. 65v. (30th Sept. 1631).
4. See above p. 51. On Jan. 21st 1632 the Town Council of Prato took notice that it was difficult to hire a surgeon because 'many members of the profession died during the epidemic' in the Grand Duchy of Tuscany (ASP, *Diurno*, 3, c. 112v.). In Milan according to Dr Tadino, almost all the surgeons and barbers died. He gives a figure of 108 deceased (TADINO, *Raguaglio*, pp. 102-3).
5. See below, Appendix 1.

ported that 'those who die here are all poor people'.[1] A similar remark was made for Florence by Rondinelli: 'the greatest part of the losses are among the poor'.[2] This was not unusual. Rightly or wrongly the plague had been always considered largely a disease of the poor and at one time it acquired the name of the beggars' disease, at another the poor's plague and at another *miseriae morbus*.[3]

In Prato, on October 7th, 1631, 'the lazaretto having been left without sick and wanting to rid it of all the rotten things', 'diligent review' was made of everything it contained. The 'bad' furnishings were burnt, while it was agreed to keep the 'florid and good' ones for 'some little while' for any eventuality. The fire that was to cancel the last traces of the tragic epidemic was started with some solemnity: the last furnishings 'were burnt on 8th November 1633 in the presence of the *Podestà* and Signor Filippo Lippi, *Provveditore* to the Illustrious Health officers of Florence'.[4] The plague was now a distant memory. The dead were at peace. And the by-standers at the bonfire no doubt congratulated themselves on still being alive.

1. ASP, *Sanità*, Negozi, b. 152, c. 1144.

2. RONDINELLI, *Contagio in Firenze*, pp. 34-36. See also CATELLACCI, *Ricordi*, p. 390.

3. SIMPSON, *Treatise*, p. 191 and CIPOLLA-ZANETTI, *Differential Mortality*.

4. ASP, LS, c. 95.

EPILOGUE

An epidemic of plague meant not only human tragedy; it also meant economic disaster. Merchants and craftsmen were those who suffered most not only because the epidemic reduced the local market but also and especially because the health restrictions paralyzed trade and communication with external markets. In the early seventeenth century however, Prato was not a major trading or manufacturing centre. The economic policy of the Grand Duke favoured the woollen industry of Florence at the expense of the industries of the minor centres. Silk was produced in Prato but mostly for Florentine merchants. The lack of major economic opportunities made administrative positions particularly sought after – such as those of '*Provveditore di Grascia*', Treasurer of the City, Governor of the Hospital, administrator of local foundations and the like.[1] Yet even in a case like Prato's, where private fortunes were not particularly vulnerable, the plague was an economic disaster for the community.

The revenue of the Community mostly consisted of duties ('*gabelle*') and the predial tithe and in the years 1626-1630 the town's treasury collected the amounts shown on p. 110 (in current *lire*).[2]

It was not a large revenue: it was no higher than the income of the hospital *della Misericordia* in years of normal agricultural prices. This was typical in pre-industrial Europe. Town and State administrations were not responsible for expenses which

1. FIUMI, *Prato*, p. 199.   2. ASP, *Fondo Comunale*, b. 587, c. 1193 ff.

	May 1626 to April 1627	May 1627 to April 1628	May 1628 to April 1629	May 1629 to April 1630	May 1630 to April 1631
Bread	12,300	12,050	11,375	11,625	11,100
Meat	4,542	4,626	3,830	3,965	4,100
Civil Justice	3,553	2,703	3,295	3,568	3,010
Wine	3,128	3,168	3,258	3,618	2,668
Weights and	578	615	668	668	458
Measures	215	238	233	238	179
Grains	970	1,005	1,060	1,080	1,030
Salt	1,591	1,638	1,596	2,100	2,200
Tithe	7,103	7,074	7,158	7,059	7,050
Others	10,893	10,160	11,707	10,927	9,113
Total	44,873	43,277	44,180	44,848	40,908
drawn from the Monte di Pietà	—	—	—	5,775	7,000

today we are accustomed to consider part of the public budget.
In Prato during the plague the town paid only part of the cost
of operation of the lazaretto and the hospital took care of the
rest. If public revenues were small, public expenses were
limited and carefully watched. In normal years the budget of
Prato showed a small surplus, as indicated by the following
figures (in current *lire*)[1]:

	revenues (lire)	expenditure (lire)	balance (lire)
1st May 1626 – 30th April 1627	44,873	44,089	+ 784
1st May 1627 – 30th April 1628	43,277	42,483	+ 794
1st May 1628 – 30th April 1629	44,180	43,485	+ 695
1st May 1629 – 30th April 1630	50,623	48,863	+1760

1. ASP, *Fondo Comunale*, b. 587, c. 1493 ff. and b. 588, c. 1202 ff.

The plague broke this delicate equilibrium. The figures on page 110 for the period May 1630 to April 1631 show that the plague caused a reduction of about 10 per cent in the town's revenues. The reduction was not greater because many *gabelle* were farmed to private collectors in order to substitute a certain for a fluctuating revenue. The administration withdrew 7,000 *lire* from the town's deposits with the *Monte di Pietà* and with this sum the budget of Prato between May 1st, 1630 and April 30th, 1631 showed an 'income' of 47,908 *lire*. Ordinary expenditures remained more or less on the same level of previous years, i.e. 46,721. Thus the 7,000 *lire* withdrawn from the *Monte di Pietà* served to fill the gap between the revenues and the ordinary outlays. The trouble was that in addition to the ordinary expenses there were large extra-expenses for Public Health caused by the contagion. According to a report by Chancellor Mainardi in which he lucidly summarized the financial situation, by January 1631 the Community was already indebted to its treasurer Ser Andrea Migliorati to the tune of 1,500 ducats (10,500 *lire*) which Migliorati had advanced out of his own pocket in order to satisfy the most urgent needs for Public Health. Chancellor Mainardi commented that it was a good fortune to have a man of means as Treasurer.[1] He was right but the advances by Migliorati were a temporary remedy, they were not a solution.

From Sept. 1630 to April 1631 the extra expenses for Public Health contracted by the Community were as shown overleaf:[2]

1. ASF, *Sanità*, Negozi, b. 155, c. 261 and 280 (5th Febr., 1631). On the advances made by Migliorati see also ASF, *Sanità*, Negozi, b. 153, c. 731 and 744 (14th Dec. 1630), c. 1038 (22nd Dec. 1630), c. 1043 (22nd Dec. 1630).
2. ASP, *Fondo Comunale*, b. 1038, c. 130v.

	lire	soldi	denari
to soldiers for acting as guards at the passes from Sept. 5th to Dec. 26th, 1630	2,599	1	8
expenses for masonry and other requirements for Public Health from August 20th, 1630 to April 30th, 1631	4,272	17	7
for subsidies to the people confined in their homes in Prato from Sept. 23rd, 1630 to April 30th, 1631	4,658	18	8
to those confined in their homes in the countryside from Dec. 24th, 1630 to April 29th, 1631[1]	922	9	4
for wages to those in the service of the Public Health from Nov. 16th, 1630 to April 18th, 1631	5,117	10	8
	17,570	17	11

This 17,570 and odd *lire* was money actually spent over the period September 1630 to April 1631. During the same period the Community also piled up a series of debts whose repayment had to be delayed; and further expenses were incurred after April.

As I said above, the treasurer, Andrea Migliorati, advanced money of his own on behalf of the Community, but there was a limit to this. As early as November 1630, the administration of Prato started requesting permission from the Grand Duke

1. The administration of Prato was requested by Florence to provide a daily ration of bread to the amount of 8 *soldi* for those who were confined in their houses outside the walls but still in territory subject to the jurisdiction of Prato (ASF, *Sanità*, Negozi, b. 153, c. 936, Dec. 12th, 1630). The administration of Prato claimed that the town was already indebted and could not assume this extra burden (ASF, *Sanità*, Negozi, b. 153, c. 1038, Dec. 22nd, 1630) but the officers in Florence insisted and won.

to draw from the deposits it had with the *Monte di Pietà* in Florence and from the funds of the *Ceppo* – the charitable foundation established centuries before by the 'Merchant of Prato'. The administration in Florence recognized the urgency of the situation and on several occasions allowed the withdrawal of funds.[1] The financial history of the Community during the late 1631 and in the following years is dominated by one leitmotiv – paying off the debts which it incurred during the epidemics.[2] I do not want to bore the reader with the details of this story, but I would like to stress two points that in my opinion throw much light on the cultural and social aspects of a pre-industrial society.

First of all it appears that during the crisis the treasury did not pay its creditors regularly. The apothecary who supplied medicines to the pest-house, a number of people who had their household wares and clothes burned because of suspected infection, the man who rented his house to the community to house the friars of St Anne[3] – all these and many others were not regularly paid at the moment of the transaction or when reimbursement or rent was due. More often than not they were just credited for the amount of money due to them. Even the salaries of those who were in the service of the Public Health were not paid regularly.[4] At the end of the epidemic the Community had an outstanding debt that it took years to pay off. The fact, however, was regarded neither as objectionable

1. ASP, *Diurno* 2, c. 167 (1st Nov. 1630); *Diurno* 3, c. 3 (28th March 1631), c. 136v. (29th April 1632), c. 156v. (18th July 1632).

2. ASP, *Diurno* 3, c. 148 (15th June 1632), c. 164v. (2nd Sept. 1632).

3. ASP, *Diurno* 3, c. 79 (29th Oct. 1631), c. 164 (2nd Sept. 1632), c. 148v. (15th June 1632).

4. ASP, *Diurno* 3, c. 148v. (15th June 1632).

nor as unusual. In pre-industrial societies mutual informal credit largely satisfied those needs which in a modern industrial society are met by the activity of formal credit institutions. No one expected to be paid on time – no one paid on time. Thus a credit structure was created that in the end helped the economy.

A second fact that appears from the documentation is this: it was commonly assumed that at the end of their period of service, the employees would be awarded a *'recognitione'* (recognition) which would consist not only of a certificate of 'well-accomplished' service but also of a certain amount of money proportionate to the importance of the service rendered. The initiative was usually taken by the person concerned who addressed a petition to the authorities for the *'recognitione'*. The authorities decided whether any *'recognitione'* was deserved and then fixed the amount. An example of a *'recognitione'* is given by the town Council resolution (Sept. 3rd, 1631) on the petition from the two community doctors – Lattanzio Magiotti and Giobatta Serrati. They had both managed to survive the epidemic and according to the minutes of the meeting of the Town Council[1]

they had applied for some recognition on account of their great toil in the time of the infection in having without distinction tended all the sick with such hardship to themselves and clear danger to their lives not only in the houses but also in the lazaretto. Considering the truth of what they declared, considering with how much charity they had performed their said offices, considering the saving made since it was not necessary to bring other doctors to Prato to tend those sick with the infection as is understood was necessary in other places, it hence appearing they deserve recognition for this, it is resolved they be paid 30 ducats each.

1. ASP, *Diurno* 3, c. 65v. (30th Sept. 1631).

One of the first '*recognitioni*' issued by the administration was that for Cristofano. About the middle of August 1631, before the pest-house was closed but when the epidemic was clearly over, Cristofano had resigned from the office of *Provveditore*. On August 24th, the Health officers in the presence of the *Podestà*:

resolved to give a token to Cristofano di Giulio Ceffini once *Provveditore della Sanità* of Prato, of how the said Cristofano carried out his charge and office as above to universal satisfaction since there were no complaints against him neither during his period of office nor after his renouncing it, having served in it divers months without provision as one of the Health officers.[1]

The motion in favour of Cristofano was approved unanimously 'with the vote of the *Signor Podestà*' and the '*recognitione*' was unreservedly encomiastic. But no money was attached to it. The position of Health officer was traditionally an honorary one and although a salary had been attached to the position of *Provveditore*, it was more symbolic than substantial being no higher than that of a gravedigger.[2] Moreover, Cristofano was a wealthy citizen and the finances of the community were in a bad state. The administrators obviously thought that a verbal '*recognitione*' would be adequate, but such thinking took no account of Cristofano's personality: he was firm, just, active, honest, civic minded but when there was money at stake he did not feel himself disqualified by mere highmindedness from competing for his share. Most certainly he was not the kind of person to be satisfied with flattering words. For months he must have hoped for some generous act on the part of the administration. When he saw that there was nothing doing, in the spring of 1632 he took up his pen and sent a petition to the administration in which he mentioned all that he had done for the Public Health Service. The administration con-

1. ASP, *Diurno* 3, c. 56.   2. See below, Appendix 1.

sidered the case and resolved on a *'recognitione'* of 24 ducats.[1]
This was good, but when it was a question of money, Cristofano was not easily put off. It was difficult for him to raise his
personal case for the third time. Thus he set on the other Health
officers to ask why none of them had received a substantial
(and for him 'substantial' meant 'monetary') reward for all the
worries, troubles, dangers, work and fatigue that they had gone
through during the epidemics while others who had done much
less had received a *'recognitione'* besides a regular salary. Cristofano could be convincing. Early in May he was able to address
a petition both 'in his name and on behalf of the other eight
Health officers'. This time the administration did not take the
matter in its stride. On May 5th, 1632 no agreement was
reached and the question was adjourned to another sitting.[2]
On the 28th it was decided to give each of the petitioners six
silver spoons and six forks for the value of 12 ducats, but this
decision was not unanimous, the *gonfaloniere* voting against.[3]

The affair of the *'recognitione'* did not tarnish the prestige of
Cristofano. To be thrifty and money-minded was not regarded as a fault in Prato and never has been: so much so that
the monument in the main square of the town is not of a saint

1. ASP *Diurno* 3, c. 126v. (5th April 1632). In this resolution, it is stated
that no salary had been paid to the *Provveditore* during his eleven months'
service. Eleven months is not the right figure. Cristofano served four
months as Health officer and eight as *Provveditore*.

When Cristofano was appointed *Provveditore*, his salary was fixed at
8 ducats a month. But alongside this resolution there is a note written in
different ink: 'salary reduced to 5 ducats a month by order of ser Lorenzo
Guicciardini Commissioner of Public Health' (ASP, *Diurno* 2, c. 176v., 11th
Dec. 1630). Lorenzo Guicciardini was the head of the Health Board in
Florence and his decision must have dismayed poor Cristofano. At any rate,
according to the resolution of April 5th, 1632 Cristofano had not yet received his small salary.

2. ASP, *Diurno* 3, c. 145v.   3. ASP, *Diurno* 3, c. 146.

or of Garibaldi, as in all other Italian cities, but of a merchant, Francesco Datini, holding in his hands a bundle of bills of exchange. In 1632 and in the following years Cristofano was accountant at the hospital *della Misericordia*[1] and in 1632 and in 1633 when another outbreak of plague seemed possible, Cristofano acted as Health officer again and as delegate to the Grand Duke for Public Health affairs. His activity and accomplishments were much praised on this occasion too, and this time at the end of his service, Cristofano was rewarded by the Community with a '*recognitione*' of 24 ducats[2] and, later, the gift of a horse.[3] However that was not the end of the story of Cristofano's request for pecuniary rewards. In 1634 or 1635 once more he petitioned the Town Council for a '*recognitione*' and this time for having supplied the Archives of the city with a copy of his *Libro della Sanità*.[4] Whether this request was met and whether other requests were made I do not know. Cristofano died in 1642.[5]

In the story of human events one occasionally encounters humble episodes, small occurrences that, though apparently insignificant, throw more light on the real character of a period than the so-called great historical events. Diacinto Gramigna was the son of the surgeon, Antonio Gramigna, who had died in October 1630. After another surgeon had died, a third one refused to treat the infected and no others could be found, Diacinto was appointed surgeon in the pest-house at the Con-

1. ASP, *Fondo Comunale*, b. 588, cc. 1043 and 1076.
2. ASP, *Fondo Comunale*, b. 227, c. 52 (22nd Sept. 1633).
3. ASP, *Fondo Comunale*, b. 227, c. 81 (3rd Febr. 1634).
4. ASP, *Fondo Comunale*, b. 588, c. 680 (undated).
5. There is a note in the *Libro dei morti* in ASP, *Fondo Comunale*, b. 3081 which says that Cristofano di Giulio Ceffini was buried in the Church of San Francesco on the 4th of July 1642. I must confess that when I read that line I felt as if I had lost an old friend.

vent of St Anne. Though he was not a qualified surgeon, he had had practical experience when helping his father. Diacinto served in the pest-house from February 16th, 1631[1] until the pest-house was closed on October 7th. On May 6th, 1632, the Town Council resolved to give Diacinto Gramigna a 'recognitione' of 15 ducats 'to have himself a suit of clothes made and burn the one he had worn while serving as Public Health surgeon'.[2] As pest-house surgeon Diacinto had served for almost eight months lancing buboes, cauterizing wounds, practising blood-letting, c tching the plague, recovering from it – and he always wore th^ same suit of clothes. As the cost of a suit almost equalled his monthly income, seven months after the pest-house had been closed, Diacinto was still wearing the same clothes. Such was the poverty of pre-industrial societies that it all but did the microbes' work for them.

If one compares the measures taken against the Black Death by Italian towns in 1348[3] with what I have described in the foregoing chapters of this book, one can see the progress that had been made in the field of Public Health over three centuries during which the plague ravaged Europe, endemically as well as epidemically. As a response to the challenge of the disease, permanent Health offices were created, permanent or temporary pest-houses were built, the use of health cordons and health passes was developed, a set of rules was worked out for quarantine and disinfection, and an elaborate network for

1. See above p. 58, n. 3.

2. ASP, Diurno 3, c. 138. In Turin, during the 1599 plague, a Frenchman and a Spaniard volunteered to serve in the pest-house on condition that the community would provide each of them with 'a new suit of clothes like the one he is wearing' (ACT, Ordinati, b. 149, c. 11, 17th June 1599).

3. For Venice see BRUNETTI, Venezia; for Tuscany, CHIAPELLI, Ordinamenti and CARABELLESE, Peste; for Orvieto CARPENTIER, Orvieto.

passing information among towns and communities was established.

In the previous chapters I persistently indicated the precise date of each measure taken and of each letter written by the officers who dealt with Public Health affairs. I did not do this under the compulsion of scholarly pedantry. Such information offers the best evidence of the remarkable promptness with which the officers took care of Public Health affairs. Letters were answered within hours of their arrival; instructions were provided without delay; commissioners were sent promptly to the points where they were needed.

The Health Board of Florence corresponded with each community of the Grand Duchy as it did with Prato. The volume of correspondence preserved in the Archivio di Stato in Florence for the years 1629-31 is good evidence of the enormous amount of work that was done. The dates of the letters are there to prove that the work was done promptly and efficiently. The officers must have spent endless hours each day of the week reading the numerous letters received, making quick decisions and pondering and dictating the answers. Behind the terse style of the correspondence, we must also imagine the worries, responsibilities, uncertainties and frustrations that piled up together with the sheer amount of work and made its load immeasurably greater. What were the results of all this dedicated activity?

The best chances of positive results were in the establishment of the external health cordon. We have a few examples of communities that during the epidemic of 1630 or during other epidemics escaped infection because of the unrelenting and inflexible vigilance exerted at the perimeter of the defences. For big cities which largely depended on trade, however, this kind of control was extremely difficult.

If and where the disease broke through the external de-

fences, the battle was lost. After the epidemic that ravaged
Genoa in 1657 killing about 55,000 out of 73,000 people, the
superintendent of the pest-house, father Antero Maria di San
Bonaventura, sceptically asked himself: 'If no measures had
been taken to rid the city of the epidemic, would Genoa have
suffered greater losses?'[1]

The officers fought against an invisible enemy. They did not
know what the enemy was, or how it struck. Medical knowledge was of no help and medical treatment was of no value.
This most officers knew. Prevention was the only hope, but it
is difficult to devise preventive measures if one does not know
the agents of infection and the way they strike. The Health
officers were working in the dark. This is shown by their
attitudes towards quarantine. For contacts the officers generally prescribed a quarantine of 22 days. This was approved by
some physicians and criticized by others who thought necessary a quarantine of at least 40 days.[2] Today we know that both
views were unnecessarily rigorous. The incubation period of
plague does not last generally more than three to five days and

1. ANTERO, *Lazzaretti*, pp. 510-11.
2. A number of physicians believed that 'ordinarily' a quarantine of
'three quarters of a moon' was adequate for contacts. (TADINO, *Raguaglio*,
p. 66). However PARISI, *Avvertimento*, p. 31, believed that 'suspects had to
be quarantined for at least forty days' and he regarded as excessively per-
missive those physicians who authorized shorter quarantines. INGRASSIA,
Informatione, vol. 1, p. 162 wrote that 'those who recommend a quarantine
of 45 days for the contacts cannot be wrong especially in winter time
when the disease remains more easily hidden'. TADINO, *Raguaglio*, p. 128
reports that in Milan in 1630 'a controversy arose about the quarantine of
forty days for the infected and twenty-two days for the contacts. It was
observed that often the contacts fell prey to the disease three or four days
after the end of their limited quarantine'. It was thus recommended (*ibid.*,
p. 66) to extend the quarantine for the contacts 'to 30 days or even to 40
days when the weather is cold'.

only exceptionally up to 14 days.[1] It is not the shortest period of incubation that is the most important for preventive measures, on the other hand the cases in which incubation appears to extend to 12 and even 14 days are rarities. The Paris Convention of 1903 fixed a period of five days for isolation of persons from plague-infected ships, which may or may not be followed by surveillance of not more than five days.[2]

The question of how long patients who have recovered from the plague remain in an infective state is more complicated. The importance of a bacteriological examination of the sputum is obvious, but as late as 1903 it could be authoritatively maintained that this question required 'more investigation than it has yet received'.[3] The Health officers of the seventeenth century with no knowledge about bacteria and bacteriological examinations, were obviously more harassed by uncomfortable uncertainty. They insisted upon a quarantine of at least forty days and they were often inclined to extend it to sixty or eighty days.

Essentially the two types of quarantines – the quarantine of at least 22 days for the contacts and the quarantine of at least 40 days for the convalescents – related to two different things. The former related to the period of incubation of the disease while the latter related to the period of infectivity of the patient. The instructions issued by the Health Board in Florence in 1630 in this regard were particularly confusing. They seemed to authorize a quarantine of 22 days for the contact as well as for the convalescent, and this was the practice followed in Prato. Most Health officers in other states and the medical profession in general would have strongly

1. SIMPSON, *Treatise on Plague*, p. 259; WU, *Plague*, p. 465; POLLITZER, *Plague*, pp. 410-11.

2. SIMPSON, *Treatise on Plague*, p. 259.

3. SIMPSON, *Treatise on Plague*, p. 258.

condemned this practice. Why the Board of Florence was so lenient with convalescents I do not know.[1] The fact remains, however, that whether the period of 22 days was adopted or that of 40 or 60 or 80, there was no scientific basis for it, everything depending on guess work. Essentially the officers' basic rule was that as far as precautions were concerned too much was obviously better than too little. But if this was the ideal, in practice their action was constantly frustrated by a number of factors outside their control. People of high rank could hardly be persuaded to submit to the rules of the officers. For totally different reasons and in a different spirit, the mass of the populace also showed little liking for discipline and obedience. We saw that in Prato it was difficult to keep even the infected people of the pest-house in complete isolation. Moreover there were often powerful vested interests that came into conflict with the needs of the Public Health. Merchants did not easily submit to those orders which forbade commercial intercourse with infected areas, and in the name of employment and prosperity they often managed to obtain exemptions that dangerously infringed the delicate defensive structure set up by the Health Boards. As was illustrated in the foregoing narrative, the individual selfishness and narrow mindedness of prominent people greatly contributed to the difficulties of the

1. The Board was not so lenient with the convalescents of the pest-house at San Miniato outside Florence. In September 1630, the Board instructed the Superintendent of the pest-house 'not to free the convalescents before a physician has certified and reported to the Board that they are safe both for themselves and for others' (ASF, *Sanità*, Copialettere, b. 55, c. 141v.-142).

In Busto Arsizio in 1630 it was decreed that for many days after their convalescence, those who had recovered from the plague 'had to carry in one of their hands a white stick three arms long so that when they went around either in town or in the countryside, they could be easily recognized and promptly avoided by other people' (JOHNSSON, *Peste in Busto Arsizio*, p. 47).

Health officers. And the latter in their turn were unconscious victims of limitations peculiar to their age. Throughout the Middle Ages and the Renaissance sharp social distinctions not only marked the boundaries among different urban classes but also sharply separated those who lived within the walls of the urban centres and those who lived outside. The latter were looked upon by the former as second-class citizens, in much the same way as the natives of the colonies were regarded by the citizens of a colonial power in the nineteenth century. When the pest-house of Prato was transferred to the convent of St Anne, the administrators of Prato were reluctant to admit the sick people from the countryside. The Board in Florence had to intervene with a strong letter in favour of the peasants and point out that it was 'in the public interest' to admit patients from the countryside into the pest-house because 'by eradicating the disease outside the walls, its eradication within is made easier'.[1]

That eminent historian of epidemics, Alfonso Corradi, lucidly summarized all these problems when he wrote that:

isolation, quarantines and purges failed in their effect because they were applied irregularly and without constant vigilance and because their purpose was not well understood, they were not supported by the cooperation of all members of society . . . Cunning, privilege and private power stood above and beyond the laws, mocking the regulations that carried extremely severe, even cruel punishments for people who were less powerful or less cunning. Quarantine within the town was of no use since its effectiveness was hindered by numerous factors, the chief one being that it was enforced in the very places where the plague had its origin. The introduction of quarantine testifies to the credit now given to the theory of contagion. The results were unsatisfactory not because the basic

1. ASF, *Sanità*, Copialettere, b. 56, c. 83 (11th Dec. 1630).

principle was mistaken but because of the enormous difficulty in putting it into practice, ignorance of the various conditions involved in the spread of infection, the ways in which this happens, the things it attaches itself to.[1]

This is the diagnosis of a great historian of medicine who was also a great physician. As an economic historian, I feel that I can add another element to the diagnosis. Besides medical ignorance and the lack of co-operation on the part of the mass of the people, the lack of adequate economic resources was perhaps the most important factor in frustrating the work of the Public Health officers. The story of Cristofano Ceffini is both pathetic and symbolic. Often he felt 'without light' lost in the darkness of an absurd fight against an invisible enemy. All too often he knew how much of his work and of the work of his colleagues was frustrated by the obstinacy, the ignorance, the stupidity, the carelessness of the people at large. But there was more to it than that. Often a chronic lack of funds and resources forced him to follow a course of action that he himself, in his deep ignorance of the enemy, intuitively felt to be tragically dangerous. Scarcity imposed choices and safety had to be sacrificed to economy.

1. CORRADI, *Annali delle epidemie*, vol. 3, p. 71.

APPENDIXES

BIBLIOGRAPHY

INDEX

PERSONNEL, WAGES AND STANDARDS OF LIVING

In the fifth section of Chapter II, we saw that the personnel engaged in combating the plague could be divided into two groups – on the one hand the physicians and surgeons who were normally to be found in Prato either employed by the town or with their own practice; on the other, those who were taken on as a special measure in time of plague. This distinction is essentially an administrative one. The 'extra' personnel were paid out of a special fund called '*della Sanità*'.[1]

I have already described the physicians and the surgeons – in Chapter II. The following notes deal with the extra personnel taken on after the epidemic had broken out. As we saw, the first death officially recognized as plague occurred in Prato on September 19th, 1630. On October 2nd, the Health officers of Prato informed the Board in Florence that the plague was spreading.[2] The same day the officers decided to turn the hospital of San Silvestro into a pest-house[3] and they hurriedly proceeded to appoint the first group of extra personnel. Significantly enough the first appointed were the gravediggers, four in number, with a monthly salary of three ducats (21 *lire*) each.[4] The gravediggers had the task not only of burying the

1. ASP, *Fondo Comunale*, b. 1038, *Entrata e Uscita del Camerlengo Generale* 1630-1, c. 130v.
2. For all this see above p. 42.   3. See above p. 46.
4. ASP, *Diurno 2*, c. 149v. (2nd Oct. 1630).

dead but also of carrying the sick from their homes to the pest-house, an arrangement which was undoubtedly practical but of dubious value for the psychological well-being of the patients. One week later, on October 9th and 10th the officers appointed the personnel for the pest-house, namely:[1]

(1) a confessor with the monthly salary of 16 ducats (112 *lire*)
(2) a surgeon, master Tiburzio Bardi, with a monthly salary of 13 ducats (91 *lire*)
(3 & 4) two attendants with the monthly salary of 8 ducats each (56 *lire* each)
(5) a man who had to deliver food and allowances to those confined in their homes, with a salary of 10 *lire* per month.

Thus by October 11th the extra personnel directly employed under the Health officers consisted of 9 people with a cost to the community of 409 *lire* per month. By October 22nd when the Chancellor of Prato wrote a report to the Health Board in Florence,[2] the situation had not changed, but things were far from being stabilized. The gravediggers refused to continue their work at the wage rate of 3 ducats per month. The officers had no choice and on October 24th they raised the wage to 30 *lire* (four ducats and 2 *lire*), which was equivalent to an increase of 42 per cent.[3] At the same time the number of patients in the pest-house went on growing and two attendants were no longer enough. The officers decided to appoint a third attendant with the same salary as the other two (8

1. The appointments were made as emergency measures on October 9th and 10th. They were registered in the minutes of the Town Council sitting of October 22nd: ASP, *Diurno* 2, c. 161.

2. ASF, *Sanità*, Negozi, b. 151, c. 1086. The man who issued the sanitary passes is not included in the list. He was underchancellor and the issuing of the passes was obviously regarded as a normal public function.

3. ASP, *Diurno* 2, c. 162.

ducats = 56 *lire* per month) and in addition another man who would carry the provisions from the hospital *della Miseri-cordia* to the pest-house. For this man the officers fixed a wage of 1 *giulio* (13 *soldi*, 4 *denari*) per day.[1] Thus by the end of October, with the exclusion of the man who issued the health passes, there were 11 people employed by the *Sanità* and the monthly expense for the community had risen to 521 *lire*. This, however, was not the end of the story.

By November 1st, three of the gravediggers had died, the fourth refused to continue his work at 30 *lire* per month and at the current wage rate it was difficult to fill the three vacant positions. Again the officers had no choice. This time they raised the salary, by 87 per cent, offering 8 ducats (56 *lire*), per month, and were able to appoint three new gravediggers.[2]

In the meantime two of the attendants in the pest-house fell sick and one died on November 2nd.[3] The officers appointed a new attendant on November 1st,[4] and a second one on November 5th,[5] both at the monthly wage of 8 ducats (56 *lire*) each. It might be supposed that the attendants were not as greedy as the gravediggers, but the gravediggers had started from a much lower rate of pay and their action was obviously aimed at obtaining a wage on a level with that of the attendants. Once they had reached that level they made no more claims.

An irreplaceable loss was that of the surgeon. On November 1st master Tiburzio Bardi died and as indicated above, despite

1. The two appointments were made respectively on October 24th and 26th but were registered in the minutes of the meeting of the Town Council of October 27th (ASP, *Diurno* 2, c. 163v.).

2. ASP, *Diurno* 2, c. 167v. (1st Nov. 1630).

3. ASP, *Diurno* 2, c. 169v. (5th Nov. 1630).

4. ASP, *Diurno* 2, c. 167v. (1st Nov. 1630).

5. ASP, *Diurno* 2, c. 169v. (5th Nov. 1630).

their desperate efforts, the officers were unable to replace him until mid-January 1631.[1]

At this juncture probably because of fear, the man who was in charge of delivering the allowances gave up the job. The officers turned his assignment over to the man who carried the victuals from the hospital *della Misericordia* to the pest-house, adding to his pay[2] 10 *lire* per month, which was the remuneration previously paid to the man who had resigned.[3]

In the midst of all these troubles, the Health officers found themselves with more and more work on their shoulders – while the citizens did not always obey their orders. So they appointed a 'runner' – a '*donzello*' – to take their messages round and generally fetch and carry; three soldiers to guard the gates of the pest-house; and two permanent guards for the two gates of the city. (The other gates were permanently closed.) For the '*donzello*' as well as for each of the three guards of the pest-house, the officers fixed a salary of 3 ducats (21 *lire*) per month while for the guards at the gates of the city they fixed a salary of 4 ducats (28 *lire*).[4]

In the meantime three more gravediggers died. On November 9th the officers replaced all three,[5] but a few days later, in view of the large number of people who had either to be buried or brought to the hospital, the officers decided that

1. See above pp. 51-2.

2. His pay was 1 giulio (*s.* 13, *d.* 4) per day equivalent to 20 *lire* for a month of thirty days.

3. ASP, *Diurno* 2, c. 168 (2nd Nov. 1630). With the addition of the 10 *lire*, the salary of this man reached 30 *lire* per month.

4. For the '*donzello*', see ASP, *Diurno* 2, c. 168 (2nd Nov. 1630). For the guards at the pest-house see ASP, *Diurno* 2, c. 171 (9th Nov. 1630). For the guards at the gates of the city, ASP, *Diurno* 2, c. 171v. (14th Nov. 1630). The Florentine officers reduced the salary of the guards at the gates from 4 ducats to 3 ducats per month.

5. ASP, *Diurno* 2, c. 171 (9th Nov. 1630).

four gravediggers were not enough. On November 12th they
appointed a fifth gravedigger with the usual monthly pay of
8 ducats.[1] By November 28th only one was alive. The same
day the officers appointed five new gravediggers. They now
numbered six, with the usual monthly pay of 8 ducats per
month.[2] Within five days one of them had already died and
had been replaced.[3] Things were not more cheerful for the
attendants in the pest-house. By November 18th, two out of
three had died and had had to be replaced.[4]

In the face of all this funereal turnover in people, wages
remained remarkably stable except the pay of the '*donzello*'
and the man who delivered the allowances. At the end of
November, the salary of the '*donzello*' was raised from 3
ducats (21 *lire*) to 30 *lire*.[5] The salary of the man who delivered
the allowances was increased from 30[6] to 49 *lire*.[7]

At this time it was also decided to give the chief constable
100 *lire* per month in addition to his regular salary in recognition of all the extra work he had to do in enforcing the
ordinances of the Health officers.[8]

Then the tide turned. On December 31st 'noticing that
thanks to God things pertaining to Public Health are improving and consequently the heavy load of work is diminishing',
the officers ordered the reduction of the additional salary of the
chief constable from 100 to 70 *lire*. The salary of the '*donzello*'
was also reduced from 30 to 20 *lire* and the salary of the man

1. ASP, *Diurno* 2, c. 171.   2. ASP, *Diurno* 2, c. 173v.
3. ASP, *Diurno* 2, c. 174 (2nd Dec. 1630).
4. ASP, *Diurno* 2, c. 172v.
5. ASP, *Diurno* 2, c. 174 (28th Nov. 1630).
6. Twenty *lire* (i.e. 1 *giulio* per day) for carrying the victuals from the
hospital *della Misericordia* to the pest-house plus ten *lire* for delivering the
allowances to the confined in their homes.
7. ASP, *Diurno* 2, c. 174 (28th Nov. 1630).
8. ASP, *Diurno* 2, c. 173v-174 (28th Nov. 1630).

who delivered the allowances from 49 to 30 *lire*.[1] On Jan. 14th, 1631, the pest-house was moved to the Convent of St Anne outside the walls of the city and the guards at the gates of the hospital of San Silvestro were also dismissed. When the new pest-house was set up outside the walls, a surgeon was appointed to it.[2] He was granted a salary of 18 ducats (126 *lire*) plus a bonus *una tantum* of 4 ducats.[3] It might be of some interest to note that when in the previous month of October the officers had made their first appointments they gave the confessor a monthly salary higher than that of the surgeon (16 against 13 ducats). Now, toward the end of the epidemic, after being deprived of the services of a surgeon for more than two months, the officers granted the surgeon a higher salary than that of the confessor – in fact, the highest salary of all.

On February 5th, 1631, Chancellor Mainardi sent to Florence the following list of those who were working for the *Sanità*:[4]

	Number	Monthly wage per person (*ducats*)
attendants in the pest-house	3	8
gravediggers	6	8
confessor	1	16
surgeon	1	18
chief constable[5]	1	10
donzello	1	3
carrier of allowances	1	4 and 2 *lire*
guards at the gates of the city	2	4
Provveditore (Cristofano)	1	8

1. ASP, *Diurno* 2, c. 182v. (31st Dec. 1630).
2. See above p. 58, n. 3.
3. ASP, *Diurno* 2, c. 184v. (13th Jan. 1631).
4. ASF, *Sanità*, Negozi, b. 155, c. 261 and 280.
5. Of course the chief constable was a regular member of the ordinary

sum total: 17 people with a cost for the community of 975 lire per month.[1] If one compares these figures with those I gave above for October 11th, 1630 (9 people = 409 *lire*) one must come to the conclusion that Parkinson's law also operates in time of plague.[2]

In the twentieth century these people would have kept their jobs and their wages till the end of their days. It is to the merit of the Tuscan administration of the time that as the plague declined, efforts were made to eliminate expenses that were becoming superfluous. I indicated above that at the very end of 1630 the salaries of three employees were reduced. On April 15th the Health Board in Florence instructed the officers in Prato to reduce the pay of the gravediggers to 5 ducats per

---

administration of the town. It is peculiar that while his additional pay for what he did for the Public Health is listed here together with the wages of the extra personnel, employed under the Health officers, one does not find in this list the additional remuneration paid to the under-chancellor ser Fausto Novellucci for the issuing of the Sanitary passes. The reason may be that the issuing of the health passes was always regarded as part of routine administration.

1. These figures do not include the women who washed clothes for the pest-house. I do not know their number, nor the kind of working relationship that they had with the community. There is no mention of this type of worker in the list by Chancellor Mainardi. Yet, on March 23rd, 1631, a woman petitioned payment of the washing she had done for the pest-house over the previous four months. She was given 8 ducats for the whole period (ASP, *Diurno* 3, c. 26). On July 1st, 1631 a new washerwoman was appointed for the pest-house with a monthly salary of 2 ducats (ASP, *Diurno* 3, c. 41).

2. In July 1631 at the peak of the plague, Padua with about 100,000 inhabitants had about 110 people employed by the Health Board (FERRARI *Ufficio Sanità*, pp. 60-1). Thus Padua had about 1 Health worker per thousand inhabitants while Prato had about three.

month (35 *lire*).[1] At the end of July the Board gave the *Podestà* further and more drastic instructions:[2]

> since the sickness has ceased in your town and there is no longer need for so many, you shall meet with the Health officers and reduce all posts and salaries – except for those serving in the pesthouse – to the number that is necessary and no more. If you proceed with the current expenses they will not be approved.

What was the real value of the wages mentioned above? We have seen that the town gave an allowance of 1 *giulio* (13 *soldi* and 4 *denari*) per day to people confined to their homes. Later, following Cristofano's appointment as *Provveditore* of Public Health (December 11th, 1630), this allowance was cut to 10 *soldi* a day. With 10 *soldi* 'they could easily sustain themselves' writes Cristofano, but knowing his parsimony, we must take the adverb 'easily' with more than a pinch of salt.

Cristofano also asserts that the daily allowance was reduced from 10 to 5 *soldi* for the poor who were getting the free bread ration. A diet in which bread alone corresponds to 50 per cent of the outlay can hardly be called rich! There are other facts that support this point. In those times in Prato, a '*staio*' (24.3 litres) of wheat gave an average 44 pounds (about 15 kilogrammes) of bread (cf. below Appendix 2). In a year of overabundant harvest when prices dropped so low as to make life difficult for the landowners, a '*staio*' of wheat cost 50 *soldi*.[3] In a normal year it cost 80 *soldi*.[4] Thus a kilo of bread cost about $5\frac{1}{3}$ *soldi* in normal years and about $3\frac{1}{3}$ *soldi* in exceptionally abund-

---

1. ASF, *Sanità*, Copialettere, b. 57, c. 68v.
2. ASF, *Sanità*, Copialettere, b. 58, c. 138v. (30th July 1631).
3. ASP, *Fondo Comunale*, b. 588, c. 194 and 217.
4. PARENTI, *Prezzi in Firenze*, p. 7 of Appendix 1.

ant ones. The reduction of the allowance from 10 to 5 *soldi* a day per person for those receiving the free bread ration shows that the administration of Prato estimated the daily average per capita consumption of bread at about one kilo. This coincides more or less with similar estimates made in other Italian towns in the sixteenth and seventeenth centuries.

If out of a daily allowance of 10 *soldi*, about 5 *soldi* were spent on one kilo of bread, what could be bought with the remaining 5 *soldi*? In abundant years a barrel of wine cost about 70 *soldi*,[1] in normal years it came to about 160 *soldi*.[2] Since one barrel contained about 46 litres, a litre thus cost $1\frac{1}{2}$ *soldi* in abundant years and $3\frac{1}{2}$ in normal ones. A daily diet of 1 kilo of bread and 1 litre of wine in a normal year therefore cost more than 8 *soldi*. With the rest one could buy some 'herbs, vinegar, oil and salt, the four substantial parts of a sallet' which, according to Robert Dallington, was 'the better part of a dinner' for most of the Tuscan population.[3]

In 1594 when prices were on average about ten per cent less than in 1630,[4] in the Inns of Florence 'he that desires to live at an ordinary, without trouble to buy his meale, vulgarly in *dozina*, shall pay for each meale two *giulii* and if he stay long, shall pay no more for two meales'.[5]

The conclusion that one can draw from all this evidence is that in Prato about 1630 an extremely poor diet cost about 10 *soldi* per day per person, which was the allowance given to the house-confinees.

1. ASP, *Fondo Comunale*, b. 588, c. 194 and 217.

2. PARENTI, *Prezzi in Firenze*, p. 11 of Appendix 1.

3. DALLINGTON, *Survey of Tuscany*, p. 55.

4. PARENTI, *Prezzi in Toscana*, p. 144.

5. MORYSON, *Itinerary* (ed. 1907), vol. 1, p. 333. Also in Pisa, Moryson 'paid upon reckoning two *giulii* for the supper and as much next day for the dinner' (*Ibid.*, p. 315). Moryson gives also the prices of individual selected commodities in Florence in 1594 (*Ibid.*, p. 333).

At the rate of 10 *soldi* per person per day, a family of four persons could not possibly have spent less than 45 *lire* (about 6 ducats) per month only for a subsistence diet. Obviously one does not live by bread alone. You need clothes, and a roof over your head. A suit of clothes for the surgeon cost some 15 ducats (105 *lire*).[1] The surgeon was superior to the manual workers but he was certainly not a member of the affluent classes; he was a typical member of the 'upper lower-class'. Naturally rents must have varied greatly. Prato gave its community's physicians an annual rent allowance of 126 *lire*, i.e. about 10 *lire* a month.[2] The doctors counted as upper class, but for the family of an artisan or a manual worker, one can hardly estimate a rent much under 1 or 2 *lire* per month.[3]

The above gives a pretty clear idea of the wretched standards of living of the time. Taking two or three *lire* for rent off the peak wage of the gravediggers or the hospital assistants (56 *lire* a month), we are left with barely enough for wine, bread and herbs for about three persons. Robert Dallington was right when he wrote:[4]

all is not gold in Italy . . . If they (the Travellers) would with me
sordida rura
atque humiles intrare casas et visere gentem
they would surely graunt that povertie and famine had not a greater kindome in those countries where Crassus starved his Armie than they have heere . . . For the poorer, their chiefest food is herbage all

1. See above p. 118.
2. See above p. 46, n. 1.
3. In 1594 in Florence 'in the *Albergo* of the Golden Keyes, called *Alle chiavi d'oro*', Fynes Moryson 'paid for my chamber by the month twelve *giulii*' (MORYSON, *Itinerary*, ed. 1907, vol. I, p. 333). Twelve *giulii* were equivalent to eight *lire*.
4. DALLINGTON, *Survey of Tuscany*, pp. 16, 31, 34.

the yeare through . . . Herbage is the most generall food of the Tuscan, at whose table a sallet is as ordinary as salt at ours . . . For every horse-load of flesh eaten, there is ten cart loades of hearbes and rootes.

Dallington quotes a conversation he had in 1596 with the Chancellor of Prato who – in Dallington's opinion – 'seemed by his discourse a man of good understanding and who ought by his office to have the knowledge hereof very familiar'. The Chancellor told Dallington that meat consumption was taxed at the rate of 5 *denari* per pound and that 'out of Prato and the precints thereof' in normal years the tax yielded about 1,000 ducats (7,000 *lire*). This meant a total consumption of above 336,000 pounds of meat per year (114,072 kilos). 'The people there being 16,000' the per capita yearly consumption of meat was about 21 pounds (7 kilos) per year: 'little more than a stone a peece for the yeare: a proportion which in Newgate market and S. Nicholas shambles will hardly be believed'.[1]

The figures quoted by Dallington are absolutely plausible. As late as the 1860's the yearly average per capita consumption of beef and pork in Italy was less than 10 kilos.[2]

Of course one has to consider that the 16,000 people mentioned by Dallington included also the infants who in pre-industrial society were relatively numerous. Moreover, the figures quoted by the Chancellor of Prato in 1596 did not take into account the meat that was produced and consumed without passing through the market, like chickens and pigeons raised in the backyards of private homes. Fish was also excluded from the calculation. All this is true, but even if we

1. DALLINGTON, *Survey of Tuscany*, p. 34.
2. ISTITUTO CENTRALE STATISTICA, *Sommario di Statistiche Storiche Italiane* 1861-1955, Rome 1958, p. 230.

were to double the average figure of 7 kilos of meat per person per year we would still remain with a very low figure, indicative both of the miserable standards of living of the mass of the population and the 'egregious and incredible parsimony' of the wealthy. In Tuscany bread, wine and salads dominated the table 'of the riche because they love to spare; of the poore, because they cannot choose; of many Religious because of their vow'.[1]

In years of normal prices, in the families of the common people, one member's work was scarcely enough to support a family of four; in one way or another wife and children had to work, even though irregularly, to bring in some extra money. Except for the privileged few, every day life consisted of a wretched routine. People were glad if they had enough food to survive on. A good solid meal was an occasion and only on special occasions could they afford such luxuries. Buying a suit of clothes was also a special event. As recounted in the epilogue, the surgeon working in the Prato pest-house wore the same clothes the entire time he spent among the infected. And he was not able to replace them when the plague finished. His monthly salary, while serving in the pest-house at the risk of his life, was 18 ducats and a new suit cost 15 ducats. Only when the Town Council presented him with extra money in

---

1. DALLINGTON, *Survey of Tuscany*, p. 34. See also the remarks made by MORYSON, *An Itinerary* (ed. 1907), vol. 4, p. 93: 'The Italians generally compared with English or French are most sparing in their diet ... Howsoever they are not so great flesh-eaters as the Northerne men, yet if the bread be weighed, which one of them eats at a meale, with a great charger full of hearbes and a little oyle mixed therein, beleeve me they have no cause to accuse Northerne men for great eaters ... (p. 96): They spend much bread and oyle ... And those that are richer do for the most part feede on bread, only they eate sallets of hearbs with their bread and mingle them with oyle.'

the form of an exceptional '*recognitione*', months after the end of his service, could the surgeon afford to throw away his old clothes. Ordinary people went around in clothes that were patched and threadbare. Few people could afford to eat well and dress well, which explains the importance that eating and dressing took on in class distinctions.

METROLOGY AND MONETARY MATTERS

The common weight used both in Florence and Prato was:

$$1 \; libbra \quad = \quad 12 \; oncie$$

When the decimal system was introduced in Tuscany a *libbra* was estimated as equivalent to $339\frac{1}{2}$ grams.

For grain the following measures were used:

$$
\begin{aligned}
1 \; moggio &= 8 \; sacchi \\
1 \; sacco &= 3 \; staia \\
1 \; staio &= 4 \; quarti
\end{aligned}
$$

The metrical equivalents of these measures are:

$$
\begin{aligned}
1 \; moggio &= 585 \; \text{litres} \\
1 \; sacco &= 73 \; \text{litres} \\
1 \; staio &= 24.3 \; \text{litres}
\end{aligned}
$$

Around 1630 it was assumed that, on average, 1 *staio* of wheat produced 44 *libbre* of bread.[1] In modern metrical equivalent, this means that 24.3 litres of wheat produced an average of about 15 kilograms of bread.

For wine the following measures were used:

1 *barile*	= 20 *fiaschi*	=	133 *libbre* and 4 ounces of liquid
1 *fiasco*	= 2 *boccali*	=	6 *libbre* and 8 ounces of liquid
1 *boccale*	= 2 *mezzetti*		
1 *mezzetto*	= 2 *quartucci*		

1. ASP, *Fondo Comunale*, b. 587, c. 1362 ff.

The metrical equivalents are:

$$1 \; barile \;\; = \;\; litres \; 45.5$$
$$1 \; fiasco \;\; = \;\; litres \;\; 2.27$$

For oil, people used units which also had the names of *barile*, *fiasco*, *boccale*, *mezzetto* and *quartuccio* but the measures were different. The *barile* for oil equalled only 16 *fiaschi* (instead of 20 as in the case of wine). For small quantities of oil the *ampolla* was also used. The breakdown of these measures was:

1 *barile*	= 16 *fiaschi*	= 90 *libbre* of liquid	
1 *fiasco*	= 2 *boccali*	= 5 *libbre* and 7 ounces of liquid	
1 *boccale*	= 2 *mezzetti*		
1 *mezzetto*	= 2 *quartucci*		
1 *boccale*	= 5.5 *ampolle*		
1 *fiasco*	= 11 *ampolle*		
1 *ampolla*	= 6 *once*		

The metrical equivalents are:

$$1 \; barile \;\; = \;\; litres \; 33.4$$
$$1 \; fiasco \;\; = \;\; about \; litres \; 2.1$$

Firewood was measured by *carrata* and *fascina*. On average 1 *carrata* was considered equivalent to 4350 *fascine*.

As to the monetary system, we have to distinguish between money of account and coins. The system of account prevailing in the first half of the seventeenth century was based on the following units and ratios:

1 *ducato* (also called *scudo*)	=	7 *lire*
1 *lira*	=	20 *soldi*
1 *soldo*	=	12 *denari*

The coins most commonly used were:[1]

name of the coin	metal	weight in grams	fineness	value in Lire	soldi	denari
doppia	gold	6.095	22 Kar	20	—	—
mezza doppia	gold	2.60	22 Kar	10	—	—
piastra	silver	22.42	958/1000	7	—	—
testone	silver	9.32	958/1000	2	—	—
lira	silver	4.65	958/1000	1	—	—
giulio	silver	3.10	958/1000	0	13	4
mezzo giulio	silver	1.55	958/1000	0	6	8
crazia	alloy	1.00		0	1	8
quattrino	copper	0.75		0	0	4

Originally the *denaro* or *picciolo* (penny) was the base and foundation of the monetary system, but owing to its progressive debasement, by the end of the fifteenth century the penny had reached such a low value that its coinage was stopped and the *denaro* survived only as a unit of account. As Dallington recorded in 1596:

There was also in times past the *denaro*, the fourth part of a *quattrino*, but now there are few of them to be seene, none to be paid. They of the country will complaine that now they have none but *moneta grossa*, great money. It was a good world say they when we might have changed a *quattrino* into 4 *denari* and with these have bought herbs, vinegar, oile and salt, the four substantial parts of a sallet and this the better part of an Italian dinner; whereas now it will cost them so many *quattrini* a great alteration, a gross sum.[2]

While the ratios among the units of account were fixed by definition, the ratios between gold and silver coins on one hand and units of account on the other could fluctuate. The

1. GALEOTTI, *Monete del Granducato*, pp. 229–90.
2. DALLINGTON, *Survey of Tuscany*, p. 55. According to Dallington a *giulio* equalled 'six-pence sterling' of English currency and a *crazia* 'the value three-farthings sterling'.

period under consideration in this book was, however, a period of monetary stability and the ratios between gold and silver coins and units of account were remarkably stable.

According to precise rules, the treasury of Prato like that of the other Tuscan town was under strict instructions to make payments in gold and silver coins and not in *quattrini*.[1]

1. ASP, *Fondo Comunale*, b. 1038. *Entrate e Uscite del Camerlengo Generale* 1630-1.

STATISTICS
ON THE PEST-HOUSE

From c. 59 to c. 63v. of his *Libro della Sanità*, Cristofano gives figures for the movement of patients as regards the pest-house at the Convent of St Anne. He provides daily figures for admissions, deaths, discharges and in-patients. I reproduce these statistics in Table 2. They cover the period from January 14th to June 16th, 1631.

The food in the pest-house was provided by the hospital *della Misericordia*, which delivered it on receipt of a '*polizza*' or delivery coupon that the *Provveditore* sent to the hospital every morning. On the coupon Cristofano marked the number of pest-house inmates who were to be fed. This explains why Cristofano had to keep a daily check on numbers in the pest-house. January 14th, 1631 was the day when the pest-house was finally in working order at the Convent of St Anne. On June 17th there were still some patients in the pest-house but for reasons we have already gone into the pest-house was put under the administration of the *Veneranda Compagnia del Pellegrino*. Thus Cristofano was freed of the job of making out the coupon for the pest-house food – and as a result no longer needed to keep up his statistics.

It is worth pointing out that in all the long series of figures given by Cristofano for the Prato pest-house one cannot find a single mistake in addition or subtraction. This may seem normal to us but it was not so normal for his times.

TABLE 2. *Admissions, deaths and discharges at the pest-house at St Anne in Prato*

	admissions	deaths	discharged convalescents	in-patients		admissions	deaths	discharged convalescents	in-patients
14 Jan.	–	–	–	43	14 Feb.	3	2	–	52
15	–	–	–	43	15	–	–	–	52
16	–	–	–	43	16	–	–	–	52
17	2	–	–	45	17	3	2	–	53
18	2	–	–	47	18	–	–	–	53
19	1	–	–	48	19	–	2	–	51
20	–	2	–	46	20	–	–	–	51
21	2	–	–	48	21	–	–	–	51
22	–	–	–	48	22	–	1	–	50
23	3	–	–	51	23	–	–	–	50
24	–	1	–	50	24	–	1	–	49
25	1	–	–	51	25	–	–	–	49
26	–	–	–	51	26	–	–	–	49
27	–	1	–	50	27	–	4	–	45
28	–	1	–	49	28	–	–	–	45
29	2	1	–	50	1 March	–	–	–	45
30	2	–	–	52	2	–	–	–	45
31	6	–	–	58	3	–	–	–	45
1 Feb.	–	1	15	42	4	–	–	–	45
2	–	1	–	41	5	–	–	–	45
3	3	–	–	44	6	2	–	–	47
4	–	1	–	43	7	3	–	–	50
5	–	–	–	43	8	2	1	–	51
6	–	–	–	43	9	2	2	–	51
7	4	1	–	46	10	–	1	–	50
8	–	2	–	44	11	5	–	–	55
9	–	1	–	43	12	–	–	11	44
10	1	–	–	44	13	1	–	–	45
11	3	3	–	44	14	2	1	–	46
12	3	1	–	46	15	–	–	–	46
13	5	–	–	51	16	1	–	–	47

	admissions	deaths	discharged convalescents	in-patients		admissions	deaths	discharged convalescents	in-patients
17 March	–	–	–	47	19 April	1	–	–	20
18	–	1	–	46	20	3	1	–	22
19	–	–	–	46	21	1	1	–	22
20	1	–	–	47	22	–	–	–	22
21	–	–	–	47	23	2	–	–	24
22	–	3	14	30	24	–	–	–	24
23	–	1	–	29	25	2	3	–	23
24	1	–	–	30	26	–	1	–	22
25	–	–	–	30	27	1	–	–	23
26	1	–	–	31	28	1	–	–	24
27	1	–	–	32	29	–	2	–	22
28	2	1	–	33	30	1	–	–	23
29	4	1	–	36	1 May	2	1	–	24
30	–	2	–	34	2	1	1	–	24
31	–	2	–	32	3	–	1	–	23
1 Apr.	2	2	–	32	4	2	–	–	25
2	–	–	7	25	5	–	–	6	19
3	1	–	–	26	6	–	–	–	19
4	–	–	–	26	7	1	–	–	20
5	1	–	–	27	8	2	1	–	21
6	1	1	–	27	9	–	2	–	19
7	–	1	–	26	10	2	–	–	21
8	–	1	–	25	11	–	2	–	19
9	–	–	–	25	12	1	–	–	20
10	–	1	–	24	13	1	1	–	20
11	2	–	–	26	14	–	1	–	19
12	2	–	–	28	15	–	–	–	19
13	–	–	9	19	16	1	–	–	20
14	2	1	–	20	17	–	1	–	19
15	1	2	–	19	18	1	–	–	20
16	1	1	–	19	19	–	–	–	20
17	2	1	–	20	20	–	1	–	19
18	–	1	–	19	21	2	–	–	21

	admissions	deaths	discharged convalescents	in-patients		admissions	deaths	discharged convalescents	in-patients
22 May	–	–	–	21	4 June	–	I	–	13
23	I	–	–	22	5	6	I	–	18
24	–	I	–	21	6	3	I	–	20
25	–	I	–	20	7	5	5	–	20
26	–	I	–	19	8	I	I	–	20
27	2	–	–	21	9	2	–	–	22
28	–	I	–	20	10	3	I	–	24
29	2	I	–	21	11	3	–	–	27
30	–	–	10	11	12	–	–	–	27
31	3	–	–	14	13	4	I	–	30
1 June	I	I	–	14	14	–	–	–	30
2	4	–	–	18	15	I	I	–	30
3	–	4	–	14	16	I	I	–	30

A comparison between the number of people who died in the lazaretto and the number of people who died in their homes must be limited to the period January 14th to May 31st because from the beginning of June also patients from the countryside were admitted to the pest-house of St Anne. The following data summarize the comparison:

	deaths in Prato	deaths in the pest-house at St Anne	total No. of deaths	deaths at St Anne as % of total
January 14th–31st	57	6	63	10
February 1st–28th	66	23	89	26
March 1st–31st	30	16	46	35
April 1st–30th	37	20	57	35
May 1st–31st	35	17	52	33
	—	—	—	—
Total	225	82	307	27

APPENDIX 4

THE FOOD IN THE PEST-HOUSE

I mentioned above in Chapter III that not only according to Cristofano but also according to other sources the patients confined in the pest-house and the convalescents confined in the '*casa del poder murato*' were not adequately provided with food, fuel and other necessities. That such complaints were not imaginary is born out by the fact that eventually the *Compagnia del Pellegrino* decided to intervene and take over the administration of both the pest-house and the convalescent-home. It is worth taking a closer look at this business.

According to the figures given by Cristofano (Appendix 3, Table 2) from January 14th to June 16th, 1631 the pest-house at the convent of St Anne had a total of 5,188 patient-days.

According to the accounts of the hospital *della Misericordia*, during the period October 1st, 1630 to June 30th, 1631 the hospital provided food for a total of 10,973 patient-days.[1] Considering that the hospital's figures cover ten months while the figures given by Ceffini cover only six months, that from October 1st to December 13th, 1630 was the worst period of the epidemic, that moreover the hospital's figures also include some infected people and their contacts who had been confined in the village of Tavola early in October 1630, there

1. ASP, *Fondo Comunale*, b. 587, cc. 1362 ff.

does not seem to be any obvious discrepancy between the hospital's figures and Ceffini's.[1]

According to the hospital's administration register, for the 10,973 patient-days, the hospital distributed:

bread	*libbre*	15,973	=	5,423 kilograms
wine	*fiaschi*	2,108	=	4,785 litres
meat	*libbre*	7,262	=	2,465 kilograms
dry grapes	*libbre*	84	=	29 kilograms
vinegar	*fiaschi*	32	=	72 litres
eggs	*no.*	1,289		
oil	*fiaschi*	24	=	50 litres
salt	*libbre*	148	=	50 kilograms
chickens		18		
beans and nuts				

It is evident that the diet in the pest-house consisted essentially of bread, meat and wine. On a basis of a total of 10,973 daily presences it can be estimated that the per capita daily consumption was:

bread about 500 grams
meat about 225 grams[2]

For reasons that I have not been able to discover wine was not offered from January 26th to March 19th, 1631 but it was given regularly during the rest of the period. If we divide the 4,785 litres consumed by the 10,973 patient-days we obtain an average of 0.436 litres per day per person, but while this

1. It is not clear however, whether the figures indicated by the hospital also included the people in the convalescent-home. The documents of the hospital mention only the pest-house.

2. According to Dr Tadino the meals served in the pest-house of Milan consisted only of bread, wine and a soup with rice and vinegar. The data supplied by the Milanese physician seem to indicate that bread was more abundantly available in the pest-house of Milan than in the pest-house of Prato but no meat was served. Cf. TADINO, *Raguaglio*, p. 67.

figure obviously does not apply for the period when the wine was not given (about two months), it underestimates the daily consumption for the period during which wine was served (about 6½ months). For the latter period, we can reasonably estimate that the daily ration must have been a little more than half a litre per day.

If the above figures are taken at their face value one would have to admit that there were enough proteins in the diet, but there was a bad deficiency in vitamins. Moreover, even if one were to suppose that for a given weight the bread of those days had a higher caloric value than today's bread, it would be difficult to maintain that the diet described above had a total value of more than 1,400–1,500 calories per man-day. This was low, especially if one considers that in the middle of the winter the patients had to live in damp rooms that were inadequately heated.

How reliable are our figures for the diet of the patients in the pest-house of St Anne? We do not know. It is difficult to imagine people surviving on a lower calorie intake than that indicated by the above calculations. On the other hand, complaints about conditions in the pest-house were so strong that the figures given above for the food supply look very rosy in comparison. It may be that not everything that left the Hospital reached the pest-house untouched. It is also true that averages mean little where daily food requirements are concerned. For about two months, no wine was served and on more than one occasion, as Cristofano recorded, the convalescents were left without a meal[1]. Last but not least, we do not know whether the number of patients who were fed as acknowledged by the hospital corresponded to the real number of people to be fed.[2]

1. See above pp. 82-3.
2. The fact that at one point the convalescents were left without a meal,

Of course, when we read the complaints about the situation in the pest-house we must consider that they represented a reaction to the cumulative effect of a minimal diet, lack of equipment (beds, blankets, mattresses, etc.), inadequate heating and lack of medicines. The latter were, objectively, of no value to say the least, but they could have offered psychological relief. As always in these cases, it is difficult to separate the subjective from the objective. Even if the figures at our disposal could be accepted at their face value, they would hardly tell us the whole story of the human tragedy.

---

seems to indicate that the hospital acknowledged its responsibility toward the patients in the pest-house but not toward the patients in the convalescent-home.

STATISTICS ON THE CONVALESCENT-HOME

At c. 64v.-66v. of his book, Cristofano gives data for the convalescent-home in the 'casa del poder murato'. The data are reproduced in Table 3. However, the convalescents also appear in two other sections of the book. The statistics that Cristofano gives on the pest-house at c. 59-63 show the number of people who were discharged from the pest-house and who allegedly had to move to the convalescents' home. The convalescents also appear in the accounts that Cristofano gives for the money he had collected from charity, because when the convalescents left the pest-house, Cristofano gave 10 *soldi* to each one of them 'until there was no money left'.

TABLE 3
Movement of convalescents at the convalescent-home

No. of admissions	Date of admission	Date of discharge	No. of days the group spent in the convalescent-home
14	Jan. 31	Feb. 8	8
5	Feb. 9	Feb. 26	17
12	Feb. 26	March 12	14
14	March 12	March 22	10
7	March 23	April 2	10
10	April 2	April 12	10
6	April 13	May 5	22
18	May 6	May 30	24
16	July 2	July 28	26
21	July 30	August 14	15

In theory those who appear as 'discharged' in the statistics for the pest-house should appear as 'admitted' in the statistics for the convalescent-home; and those who appear as 'discharged' from the convalescent-home should appear in the account of the subsidies paid by Cristofano. In fact there is a perfect correspondence between the statistics on the convalescent-home and the account of the subsidies for the period from February 8th to May 5th. After this things become confused. There were 18 discharged from the convalescent-home on May 30th but one does not find any payment of subsidies that day. On the other hand one finds that subsidies were paid to 7 convalescents on June 28th and again to 10 convalescents on July 23rd. There were 16 discharged from the convalescent-home on July 28th: the following day only 6 subsidies were paid. The reason for these inconsistencies are not difficult to imagine. By the end of June the funds in the hands of Cristofano were practically exhausted. He himself explains that the subsidies were paid regularly 'until there was no money left'. When no more money was available and he had to advance the money from his own pocket, he apparently paid the subsidies very late – and only after repeated requests from those concerned. Probably he never gave any subsidy to some of the claimants.

The statistics on the pest-house and the statistics on the convalescent-home rarely agree. The two sets of conflicting figures are shown on p. 154.

The differences of a day in the date are not very important – they may depend on book-keeping requirements. If a convalescent left the pest-house on the evening of a given day, he would, as far as concerns feeding, be found in the convalescent-home list the day after.

As regards discrepancies among the convalescent-numbers, if the number of the discharged from the pest-house is higher

| | number of convalescents | |
	discharged from the pest-houses	admitted to the convalescent-home
Jan. 31	—	14
Feb. 1	15	—
Feb. 9	—	5
Feb. 26	—	12
March 12	11	14
March 22	14	—
March 23	—	7
April 2	7	10
April 13	9	6
May 5	6	—
May 6	—	18
May 30	10	—

than that of those admitted into the convalescent-home, the difference is once again not difficult to explain. We know that a number of people were detained in the pest-house after their recovery because there was no money to provide them with new clothes. It is understandable that, if they were detained in the pest-house for a longer time than necessary, when they were discharged they were sent directly to their homes. On the other hand, we know that at times the situation at the convalescent-home was very critical because of lack of food, and it is not difficult to imagine that Cristofano when discharging people from the pest-house occasionally sent some straight back to their homes.

At times, however, the figures show that those admitted into the convalescent-homes were more numerous than those discharged from the pest-house. One possible hypothesis is that these were people who had spent the period of sickness in their homes because there was no room for them in the pest-house.

I do not think that these apparent contradictions lessen the value of Cristofano's statistics. They are to be taken as evidence, rather, of the thousand difficulties poor Cristofano had continually to cope with if he was in some way to arrange things for the sick and the convalescent – by resorting frequently to expedients that were not always orthodox.

ABOUT THE HOUSES
CLOSED IN PRATO

In his book, Cristofano gives statistics for the houses that were closed in Prato because there had been cases of infection in them, whether terminating in death or not. His statistics can be divided into two parts. In the first (c. 1-18) he gives figures for the houses that he found 'closed' when he was appointed *Provveditore* and that were 'opened' after his appointment. In the second part (c. 19-28) he gives the figures for the houses that were 'closed' after his appointment.

When he was appointed *Provveditore* on December 11th, 1630, according to his figures there were in Prato, 77 houses closed, with 223 persons confined within them. As already mentioned, it seems that some of these houses had been 'closed' for more than 22 days and this was an abuse. Cristofano immediately proceeded to open them as soon as they had terminated the period of quarantine, or if they had already gone beyond it. Table 4 summarizes Cristofano's data.

TABLE 4

Houses 'opened' by the Provveditore *from December 11th, 1630 to January 18th, 1631*

Date	No. of houses 'opened'	No. of people living in the houses
11 Dec 1630	13	35
15	9	27
20	10	31

Date	No. of houses opened	No. of people living in the house
21 Dec 1630	9	24
22	6	22
24	2	4
27	3	4
29	7	24
2 Jan 1631	4	7
3	4	13
6	1	4
7	2	5
8	1	3
9	2	8
10	1	2
12	1	3
16	1	5
18	1	2
Total	77	223

The distribution of the households in question according to the number of people confined in them was as follows:

No. of people confined within the household	No. of households
1	10
2	23
3	21
4	12
5	10
6	1

From the above it follows that the average number of people confined in the houses was 3.2; the median was 3; the modal value 2. While considering these figures the reader ought to keep in mind that many of the households in question had either suffered deaths because of the epidemic or some member of the household had been removed to the pest-house – these being the reasons for closing them. The average size of the household and the distribution of the households according to size is therefore distorted by the epidemic. Still, one is left with the impression that the average size of the household in Prato was relatively small.[1]

From December 11th, 1630 for about one month, Cristofano did nothing but 'open' houses. On January 11th he started closing others. His reason for keeping a detailed account of the houses that were shut up and of the people confined in them was essentially financial. Cristofano had to send the allowance to the confined people and consequently he had to know their number exactly. After his appointment as *Provveditore* however, it was decided not to give the subsidy to those who had enough to provide for themselves or to those who being infected refused to go to the pest-house.[2] Consequently, Cristofano, although listing all the houses that were closed, gives the number of the people who were confined in them only for households that received the allowance. His figures are summarized in Table 5.

1. In Padua on May 18th, 1631 the number of houses closed was 137 and the number of people confined in them was 771 with an average of 5.6 persons per house (FERRARI, *Ufficio della Sanità*, p. 128). Of course, it may well be that the buildings in Padua were, on average, larger than those in Prato and thus contained more families. But this is mere speculation.

2. See above pp. 78-9.

TABLE 5

Number of households closed from January 11th, 1631 to October 24th 1631[1]

| Period | No. of houses closed | | Total | No. of people con-fined in the houses that received the allowance |
	receiving the allowance	not receiving the allowance		
11-31 Jan. 1631	23	2	25	73
1-28 Feb.	13	9	22	54
1-31 March	16	5	21	51
1-30 April	17	5	22	53
1-31 May	16	4	20	40
1-30 June	20	1	21	54
Total (partial)	105	26	131	325
1-31 July	7	1	8	24
1-31 August	3	0	3	5
1-30 Sept.	1	1	2	5
1-24 Oct.	4	1	5	20
Total	120	29	149	379

The distribution of the 120 houses that received the allowance according to the number of people confined in them, was as follows:

No. of people confined in the household	No. of households
1	17
2	36
3	23
4	25

1. About the middle of August 1631, Cristofano left the post of *Provveditore*. In his book, however, he gives figures for the houses that were closed until October 24th. In this Table I give a partial total at the end of June because the epidemic practically ended then.

No. of people confined in the household	No. of households
5	7
6	6
7	4
8	—
9	—
10	I
11	I

From the above it follows that the average number of people confined in the 120 households was 3.2; the median was 3; the modal value was 2. These are exactly the same values obtained for the houses that were opened by Cristofano from December 11th, 1630 to January 18th, 1631. For these values again, we must remember that they reflect the impact of the plague on the number in the household.

When a house was closed, it did not mean that all the troubles for those confined inside were over. The source of infection in the form of infected rats or fleas was generally still there and/or infection might already have been passed on to other members of the households. Some data from Cristofano may serve to illustrate the point. On January 14th, Cristofano had two houses closed with seven people in them. One of these people was crossed out on January 25th, and another four on February 2nd. They obviously died on these dates. On January 20th, 1631, two houses were shut up with seven people confined in them. On January 28th one of these poor wretches was sent to the pest-house and on February 3rd the other six went the same way. To say that a house was 'plagued' was not a purely literary expression.

The proportion of houses that received an allowance out of the total number of houses that were closed is high (120 out of 149). This does not mean that most of the people were poor, even by the standards of those days. It simply means that about eighty per cent of the people lived on their daily working incomes and that they did not have either substantial savings or other sources of income besides their work.

If one adds the number of houses that Cristofano found closed when he was appointed *Provveditore* (77 households) to the 131 (105 with allowance plus 26 without) that he closed during the period of the epidemics (until the end of June 1631) one obtains a total of 208.

According to Cristofano some of the 77 houses that he found closed had been in quarantine for more than 22 days. We can assume that the total of 208 houses covers the period from mid-November to the end of June. During this period the number of deaths in the town totalled 707, to which one should add another 100 deaths that occurred in the pest-house outside the walls at the convent of St Anne. Dividing the number of deaths by the number of houses that were closed one obtains an average of 3.9 deaths for each house. In the light of what has been said above about the relatively small size of Prato households[1] and considering that not all those who fell ill died, the average of 3.9 deaths for each house looks too high.

It may be that:

(a) there were deceased people who were counted in the total number of deaths, but whose death was not related to the confining of a household. This would be the case of friars and nuns who were very numerous in Prato, and also of such people as beggars and the like;

(b) in the case of very small households made up of only one or two people, the whole household may have succumbed to the first attack of the plague. In this case while there was a net addition to the number of deaths, there was no reason

1. Besides what has been said above, see also FIUMI, *Prato*, p. 179.

for Cristofano to count the household among the houses that were closed since no person was confined in it.

All these, however, are hypotheses and there is no evidence to test the possible validity of any one of them.

It would be interesting to estimate the ratio of those who were quarantined in their homes to those who were quarantined in the pest-house at St Anne, but the calculation is not feasible. A number of those who were quarantined in their homes were later on moved to the pest-house. There is therefore duplication in the two sets of data and as we have no nominative lists it is impossible to identify the cases of duplication.

ON MORTALITY IN PRATO

On cc. 67v.–82 of his book, Cristofano gives the daily number of deaths that occurred within the walls of Prato from October 1st, 1630 to November 30th, 1631. The monthly totals are as follows:

October 1630	368
November	317
December	213
January 1631	110
February	66
March	30
April	37
May	35
June	37
July	5
August	4
September	3
October	6
November	5
Total	1,236

Since in the town the epidemic was over by the end of June, in the following Table 6 I have reproduced the daily figures only for the period from October 1st, 1630 to June 30th, 1631. The figures do not include those who died in the pest-house outside the walls at the convent of St Anne. This is clear from

TABLE 6

Number of deaths in Prato from October 1st, 1630 to June 30th, 1631

Day	Oct.	Nov.	Dec.	Jan.	Feb.	March	April	May	June
1	6	5	6	2	2	1	5	1	2
2	12	6	3	–	2	1	–	1	3
3	24	8	15	4	1	2	–	1	–
4	7	6	6	6	6	1	–	1	4
5	8	–	9	8	3	2	–	1	2
6	17	11	2	–	1	–	1	–	1
7	13	22	14	7	3	2	1	–	3
8	14	16	10	–	6	1	1	1	2
9	10	10	3	10	2	2	–	2	–
10	11	13	10	3	2	–	5	2	1
11	2	15	4	2	5	–	2	2	–
12	6	1	14	6	3	–	1	–	2
13	15	2	10	5	2	–	2	1	2
14	12	10	16	3	3	1	–	1	3
15	14	13	7	9	1	–	2	–	–
16	13	17	–	5	1	2	1	2	1
17	4	14	11	6	3	–	3	2	1
18	19	13	3	4	1	2	1	–	3
19	15	15	–	1	3	–	1	1	–
20	14	9	10	2	–	1	–	1	1
21	15	7	12	2	2	–	1	–	2
22	8	10	4	3	2	3	1	1	–
23	21	11	2	1	2	2	2	3	2
24	8	11	1	2	5	–	2	1	2
25	10	10	3	3	2	1	1	–	–
26	13	15	2	2	–	–	1	1	–
27	18	14	9	2	–	1	–	1	–
28	16	9	13	3	3	2	1	2	–
29	3	10	9	6	–	–	1	4	–
30	9	14	3	1	–	2	1	2	–
31	11	–	2	2	–	1	–	–	–
Total	368	317	213	110	66	30	37	35	37

the fact that on some days in which no death is indicated for the town, there were deaths in the pest-house.[1]

The ratio of those who died in the pest-house to those who died in town was reported above in Appendix 3.

1. See 27th Feb., 10th, 29th and 31st March, 14th, 20th, 25th, 29th April, 25th May, 3rd, 7th and 15th June.

APPENDIX 8

INSTRUCTIONS OF THE PUBLIC HEALTH BOARD IN FLORENCE FOR JUSTICES IN THE COUNTRYSIDE

In 1630, when the plague epidemic was raging, the central administration of the Grand Duchy of Tuscany printed: 'The Instructions of the Health Board of Florence for the Justices in the countryside in case of infectious sicknesses that might be discovered in the areas under their jurisdiction'.[1] These 'Istruzioni' were to serve as a guide for the local administrators in the countryside in combating the epidemic of plague. Since they concern the country and not the town, the instructions continually refer to peasants and tenants. They do, however, give a clear idea of the kind of instructions issued by the Central Health Board of Florence.

It being the task of all justices, criminal as well as civil, to watch over everything that concerns good government, they shall in

1. A copy of these 'Istruzioni' is preserved in ASF, Sanità, Bandi t. 2, c. 64. For comparison with general instructions in other States, see the Regole politiche in tempi di male contagioso (29th June, 1630), in ACT, Collezione IV, n. 8, Istruzioni sanitarie 1595-1852, c. 666-7, and the Istruzioni del Magistrato sopra la Sanità (30th Dec. 1630), Ibid., c. 686.

particular, above all else, have an eye to good regulations regarding the interests of the Public Health, and for this purpose shall make shift to have notice of all cases of sickness believed to be infectious that should chance in their jurisdictions and as soon as they come by news of any case whether of sickness or death, they shall observe the following and proceed to carry out the orders herein described against any persons whatsoever, even if they should be Florentine citizens or others in other ways privileged.

First, they shall give orders to whomever is concerned that those dead of suspected plague are not to be buried in the churches but in the countryside far from the high roads, and a hundred armslengths from the houses, and in a grave at least three armslengths deep with the benediction that will seem fit to the priests of the parish church where such deaths may be, and if there are no gravediggers, have the corpse put on a ladder and handling it as little as possible, carried to the grave, and, where possible, put on the said corpse lime and then earth.

As soon as the news arrives of the sickness being discovered in whatsoever house, the Justice shall give orders that the sick man be carried to the pest-house, if it is near enough for him to be carried there.

Then he will have orders given to the occupants of the house where the sickness has been, if they are tenants, that they must not leave the house and the fields where they are, that they must not associate with anybody, and must not give away anything from their house or fields under pain, for transgressors, of their lives and confiscation of their goods.

If the sick of the said houses should be far from the pest-houses so that they could not with ease be carried thither, give in any case orders that none must leave home or fields, as above, being tenants.

If the said sick are subtenants or live in houses without land the order must be given, with the said penalty, not to leave the house, to all the occupants.

As the said persons under orders need to be sustained with victuals, if they are tenants, give orders to the owners of the land that they supply the said victuals as giving them credit to repay at the harvests or in some other way.

If they are farmworkers, or occupants of houses without land, or poor, give order to the Chamberlain of the Council that he supply them with the necessary victuals from some innkeeper or shopkeeper nearby to the amount of eight *soldi* a day per head.

If the owners of the said sick tenants should not live in the same jurisdiction so that the order cannot be given to them, then have the Chamberlain of the Council supply the said expenses for victuals for the said eight *soldi* a day for each one of those under orders as above.

And they shall give orders that the victuals be brought to those under orders, not in money but in bread and eatables by the nearest innkeepers or shopkeepers or others they deem suitable, and such things should be delivered through the windows or in some other way such that whoever brings them does not approach and does not converse with the suspect cases and those under orders and for this debt they must be reimbursed by the owners of the land who in turn shall reimburse themselves from the peasants on whom the money is being spent.

The said Justices will give order to the Health Deputies nearest the dwelling of the suspects, or to other of their officials, who will from time to time go and inspect the affected areas and ensure that victuals are supplied them as above and that they do not leave the house and land respectively assigned to them as the place of disinfection, which they must do, proceeding against transgressors with every rigour, having them isolated and the doors of their houses nailed up; and then after the usual disinfection have them put into prison and advise the Magistrate of the Health Board of Florence and await orders from him which will be given.

The quarantine and disinfection that are to be carried out in each house must be of twenty-two days at least from the day that the last person sick with the suspect sickness had died or recovered; after this period the said houses can be opened and freed.

It must be noted that before the houses closed or under orders are opened even where none of the occupants is left, it is very fitting and necessary that first the said houses be perfumed and purified in the following manner and with the diligence described, that is . . .

First, whoever enters the house to perfume it should carry in his hand brushwood or something like it lighted and burning and should go upstairs with it and make fire with flames in the rooms. Then shut the windows tight and make smoke with sulphur all through the house.

Sweep the floors, benches and walls well, and if possible, white-wash the house or at least, wash the walls down with alkaline solution using a whitewashing brush. The woodwork should also be washed down with alkaline solution. Put the linen cloths to soak in water and wash the mattresses and put other cloths where they can get air, and keep them aired for many, many days before they are used again. And those that were used directly by the infected person are to be burnt if they be woollens or linen. The room where the dead or sick person had been must, for three days after it has come empty, be washed out with vinegar, and have it swept thoroughly every day, and the first time, scatter lime around the room and throw vinegar over it until it has smoked and burnt itself out.

And since it often chances that the sick are peasants far away from lands and castles and from the advantage of being able to have physicians and medicines, make very sure that they know of some easy medicines proposed to the Magistrates of the Health Board as being easy by their physicians, with which the occupants of the said houses under orders and the sick themselves may make their own medicines.

And they shall do their utmost to save those, above all, who are healthy in the said closed houses; and for this purpose the latter, every morning, shall take some Venice treacle, oil themselves with oil against the poison and other like preservatives, and if they have none of these, shall take nuts, and dried figs, and rue and, early in the morning, eat them or other things that are meant for the purpose.

Every morning the sick shall take a five-ounce glass of very hot chickpea or goat's-rue juice, and shall cover themselves well so as to sweat; they must be informed that sweating is an excellent remedy for the infectious sickness that is latent. That they strive to bring out this sweat, however, with fire or with putting cloths on or as best they can.

Oil the swellings that appear with oil of white lilies or of camomile or flax seeds and place a little wool soaked in one of these oils upon them.

If these swellings do not come out, go about to make them do so with a cupping glass or by putting white onion roasted on the embers and mixed with Venice treacle on them.

If a blister or small carbuncle be found, put devil's-bit scabious grass crushed between two stones upon it, and to remove the scab, put a little chicken fat on it and slit it with a razor and then put a little Venice treacle on it. Around the small carbuncle put pomegranate juice together with the pomegranate seeds and peel all well crushed together.

The sick must take good care of themselves and eat meat, eggs and good things; they must abstain from wine and drink boiled water with the soft part of a loaf and a few coriander seeds in it.

Note must be taken of these medicines for the use of those who cannot have, as above, the services of physicians and other medicines, those, that is, like the poor peasants who live in the countryside, etc.

BIBLIOGRAPHY

ABRATE, M., Popolazione e peste del 1630 a Carmagnola, in *Studi Piemontesi* I (Torino, 1972).

AGNELLI, G., *I lanzichenecchi e la peste del 1630 nel Lodigiano*. Lodi, 1886.

ALESSIO, A., *Preservatione della peste e historia della peste di Este*. Padova, 1660.

ANTERO, M. DA SAN BONAVENTURA, *Li Lazzaretti della Città e Riviere di Genova del MDCLVII*. Genova, 1658.

BARBATO, B., *Il Contagio di Padova nell'anno 1631*. Rovigo, 1640.

BATTARA, P., *La popolazione di Firenze alla metà del 500*. Firenze, 1935.

BATTISTINI, M., *Le epidemie in Volterra dal 1004 al 1800 con notizie particolari della peste del 1631 nei pressi vicini a Volterra, in Pisa e nel territorio Pisano*. Volterra, 1916.

BELLENTANI, P., Dialogo della peste in G. MUELLER, (ed.), *Raccolta di Cronisti Lombardi*, Milano, 1857.

BELOCH, K. J., *Bevölkerungsgeschichte Italiens*. Berlin, 1930-61.

BELTRAMI, L., *Il lazzaretto di Milano*. Milano, 1899.

BEMBO, A., Relazione della peste di Brescia fatta alla Signoria di Venezia, in ROMANIN, *Storia documentata*, vol. 7.

BENAGLIO, M. A., Relazione della carestia e della peste di Bergamo e suo territorio negli anni 1629 e 1630, in *Miscellanea di Storia Italiana*, vol. 3. Torino, 1865.

BESTA, B., La popolazione di Milano nel periodo della dominazione Spagnola, in *Atti del Convegno Internazionale per gli studi sulla popolazione*. Roma, 1933, vol. I.

BIAGETTI, L., *Alcune notizie storiche e biografiche sulla peste degli anni 1630-31-33 in Toscana*. S. Agnello di Sorrento, 1884.

BOGNETTI, G. P., Il lazzaretto di Milano e la peste del 1630, in *Archivio Storico Lombardo*, serie 5, vol. 50 (1923).

BONALDI, P. A., *Discorso razionale contro la presente epidemia pestilente*. Treviso, 1630.

BONI, G., La peste nelle Giudicarie, in *Studi Trentini*, 1922.

BORTOLAN, D., *La peste nel 1630 a Vicenza*. Venezia, 1894.

BOTTERO, A., La peste in Milano nel 1399-1400 e l'opera di Gian Galeazzo, in *Atti e Mem. dell'Accademia di Storia dell'Arte Sanitaria*, 8 (1942).

BRIGHETTI, A., *Bologna e la peste del 1630*. Bologna, 1968.

BRIGHETTI, A., La peste del 1630 a Novellara, in *Civiltà Mantovana*, 15 (1968).

BRUNETTI, M., Venezia durante la peste del 1348, in *Ateneo Veneto*, 32 (1909).

CAFFAROTTO, T. M., *Il flagello nero*. Saluzzo, 1967.

CAPASSO, G., L'officio della sanità di Monza durante la peste degli anni 1576-77, in *Archivio Storico Lombardo*, 33 (1906).

CAPPELLI, A., *Cronologia, Cronografia e Calendario Perpetuo*. Milano, 1930.

CARABELLESE, E., *La peste del 1348 e le condizioni della sanità pubblica in Toscana*. Rocca San Casciano, 1897.

CARPENTIER, E., *Une ville devant la peste. Orvieto et la Peste Noire de 1348*. Paris, 1962.

CASA, E., La peste bubbonica in Parma nell'anno 1630, in *Arch. Stor. Province Parmensi*, IV (1895).

CASTRO da, S. R., *Il curioso nel quale in dialogo si discorre del male di peste*. Pisa, 1631.

CATELLACCI, D. (ed.), Curiosi ricordi del contagio di Firenze del 1630, in *Archivio Storico Italiano*. ser. 5, vol. 20 (1897).

CAVALLINI, M., *La peste del 1631 in Volterra*. Volterra, 1915.

CENTORIO, A., *I Cinque libri degl'avvertimenti, ordini, gride et editti fatti et osservati in Milano ne' tempi sospettosi della peste gli anni 1576 et 77*. Venezia, 1579.

CHIAPPELLI, A., Gli ordinamenti sanitari del Comune di Pistoia contro la pestilenza del 1348, in *Archivio Storico Italiano*, ser. 4, vol. 20 (1887), pp. 3-24.

CIPOLLA, C. M. and ZANETTI, D., Plague and differential mortality, in *Annales d'histoire demographique*, 1972.

CLARETTA, G., *Il municipio di Torino ai tempi della pestilenza del 1630*. Torino, 1869.

COLNAT, A., *Les épidemies et l'histoire*. Paris, 1937.

CONSOLI FIEGO, G., *Peste e carestie in Pistoia*. Pistoia, 1920.

CORRADI, A., *Annali delle epidemie occorse in Italia, dalle prime memorie fino al 1850*. Bologna, 1867-1892.

CREIGHTON, C., *A History of Epidemics in Britain*. Cambridge, 1891-4.

CRINO', A. M., Documenti relativi al libro di Sir Robert Dallington sulla Toscana, in *Fatti e Figure del Seicento Anglo Toscano*, Firenze 1957.

DALLINGTON, R., *Survey of Tuscany*. London, 1605.

D'ANDREA, G., *I Riformati napoletani durante la peste del 1656*. Napoli, 1861.

DEL GUERRA, G., *Pisa attraverso i secoli*. Pisa (on pp. 258-63 it reproduces the part of a ms. by Arrosti which concerns the plague of 1630).

DE SAINT GENIS, V., *Histoire de Savoie*. Chambery, 1868.

DOLFIN, P., *Della peste. Opinioni dei medici di Venezia nel 1630*. Padova, 1843.

DUCCO, A., La peste del 1630, in P. GUERRINI, *Cronache Bresciane Inedite*, vol. 4, Brescia, 1922.

FABRONI, F., *De origine et causis pestilentis morbi anno 1630 Italiam infestantis.* Bologna, 1631.

FANO, C., *La peste bubbonica a Reggio Emilia negli anni 1630-31*. Bologna, 1908.

FEROCI, A., *La peste bubbonica in Pisa nel Medio Evo e nel 1630*. Pisa, 1893.

FERRARI, C., Il Lazzaretto di Verona e il gran contagio del 1630 in *Lettura*, 3 (1903).

FERRARI, C., Proibizioni e Trasgressioni sanitarie a Padova, in *Bollettino del Museo Civico di Padova*, 7 (1904).

FERRARI, C., Il Lazzaretto di Padova durante la peste del 1630-31 in *Bollettino del Museo Civico di Padova*, 7 (1904).

FERRARI, C., Il Censimento della Popolazione del Territorio Veronese dopo la peste del 1630, in *Atti dell'Accademia d'Agricoltura, Scienze . . . di Verona*, Serie 4, vol. 5 (1904).

FERRARI, C., L'Ufficio della Sanità in Padova nella prima metà del secolo XVII, in *Miscellanea di Storia Veneta-R. Deputazione di Storia Patria*, ser. 3, vol. I (Venezia, 1910).

FIOCHETTO, G. F., *Trattato della peste o sia contagio di Torino dell'anno 1630*. I edit. Torino 1631 (Tisma); 2 edit. Torino 1720 (Zappata). (Quotations in this book refer to the second edition.)

FIORENTINI, F. M., Relazione inedita ai Conservatori di Sanità intorno alla peste (del 1630), in G. SFORZA, *Di Francesco M. Fiorentini*, Lucca 1879.

FIUMI, E., *Demografia, movimento urbanistico e classi sociali in Prato*. Firenze, 1968.

FIUMI, L., La peste di Napoli del 1656 secondo il carteggio inedito della Nunziatura Pontificia in *Studi e documenti di Storia e diritto*, 16 (1895).

FRARI, A. A., *Della Peste e della Amministrazione Sanitaria*. Venezia, 1840.

GALASSI, N., *Dieci secoli di storia ospitaliera a Imola*. Imola, 1966-70.

GALEOTTI, A., *Le monete del Granducato di Toscana*. Livorno, 1929.

GALILEI, G., *Opere*, ed. A. Favaro. Firenze, 1909.

GALLUZZI, R., *Istoria del Granducato di Toscana*. Firenze, 1781.

GAROFALO, F., La difesa di Roma e dello Stato Pontificio contro la peste dal 1629 al 1632, in *Humana Studia*, Suppl. to n. 6 (1949).

GASTALDI, H., *Tractatus de avertenda et profliganda peste*. Bologna, 1684.

GERBALDO, G. G., Memorie della guerra, carestia e peste del Piemonte negli anni 1629, 1630 e 1631, in *Miscellanea di Storia Italiana*, vol. 5 (1868).

GHIRARDELLI, L., *Il memorando contagio seguito in Bergamo l'anno 1630*. Bergamo, 1681.

GHIRON, I., Documenti ad illustrazione dei Promessi Sposi, in *Archivio Storico Lombardo*, 5 (1878).

GIANI, G., Le pestilenze del 1348, del 1526 e del 1631-2 in Prato, in *Archivio Storico Pratese*, 9 (1930) (this work has been published after author's death and is full of mistakes).

GRILLOT, J., *Lyon affligé de contagion depuis le mois d'aôut de l'an 1628 jusqu'au mois d'octobre de l'an 1629*, Lyon, 1629.

HENSCHEN, F., *The history of diseases*. London, 1966.

HIRST, L. F., *The Conquest of Plague*. Oxford, 1953.

HOLLINGSWORTH, M. F. and T. H., Plague Mortality Rates . . . in the Parish of St Botolph's, London 1603, in *Population Studies*, 25 (1971).

HOWARD, J., *The Principal Lazzarettos in Europe*. London, 1789.

IMPERIALI, G., *Pestis anni MDCXXX historico-medica narratio*. Vicenza, 1631.

INGRASSIA, G. F., *Informatione del pestifero et contagioso morbo il quale affligge et have afflitto questa città di Palermo*. Palermo, 1576.

JETTER, D., Das Isolierungsprinzip in der Pestbekämpfung des 17 Jahrunderts, in *M.H.J.*, 5 (1970).

JOHNSSON, J. W. S., (ed.), *Storia della peste avvenuta nel borgo di Busto Arsizio 1630*, Copenhagen, 1924.

LA CAVA, A. F., *La peste di S. Carlo*. Milano, 1945.

LA CROCE, P., *Memorie delle cose notabili successe in Milano intorno al mal contaggioso l'anno 1630*. Milano, 1730.

LAMPUGNANO, A., *La pestilenza seguita in Milano l'anno 1630*. Milano, 1630.

LATRONICO, N., Una grida per il rispetto dei ministri della Sanità di Milano durante la peste del 1630, in *Le forze sanitarie* 8 (Roma, 1939).

LOCATELLI, G. B., *Della peste*. Rovigo, 1631.

MACCOLINI, R., Bologna e le grandi pandemie dei secoli passati, in *Bullettino delle Scienze Mediche*, 1940.

MAFFEI, A., *Sondrio nel 1634. Aggiunti alcuni cenni sulla pestilenza del 1630.* Sondrio, 1874.

MAGGIORE-PERNI, FR., *Palermo e le sue grandi epidemie dal secolo XVI al XIX.* Palermo, 1894.

MARIONI, P. A., (observer of the Republic of Venice in Milan), Peste in Milano nel 1630, in F. MUTINELLI, *Storia arcana ed anedottica d'Italia*, Venezia 1855-8, vol. 4, pp. 34 ff.

MASSARI, C., *Saggio storico medico sulle pestilenze di Perugia e sul governo sanitario di esse dal secolo XIV fino ai giorni nostri.* Perugia, 1838.

MAZZOLDI, L., Gli ultimi secoli del Dominio Veneto, in *Storia di Brescia*, vol. 3, Brescia, 1964.

MAZZOLDI, L., R. GIUSTI, R. SALVADORI, *Mantova. La Storia*, vol. 3. Mantova, 1963.

MEASSO, A., Carestia e febbre maligna in tempi di peste. Consulti e provvedimenti a Udine negli anni 1629-1630, in *Atti dell'Accademia di Udine*, serie 2, vol. 8 (1888).

Memorie di quanto si è fatto per preservatione della Peste a Ferrara durante il governo dell'Em. e Rev. Sig. Cardinale Sacchetti negli anni 1629, 1630 e 1631. Ferrara 1631.

MINGHETTI, R., I Lazzaretti del Seicento e loro regolamenti per la disciplina dei ricoverati e del personale addetto, in *Atti del I Congresso Europeo di Storia Ospitaliera* (Reggio Emilia, 1960), 1962.

MOLMENTI, P., *La Storia di Venezia nella vita privata*, Bergamo, 1906.

MONTINI, G. M., *Della peste in Bassano nel 1631. Narrazione inedita.* Bassano, 1856.

MONTU, G. B., *Memorie Storiche del gran contagio in Piemonte negli anni 1630 e 1631.* Torino, 1830.

MORANDO, B., *La peste di Piacenza nel 1630.* Piacenza, 1867.

MORATTI, P., *Racconto de gli ordini e provisioni fatte ne lazzaretti in Bologna e suo contado in tempo del contagio dell'anno 1630.* Bologna, 1631.

MORYSON, F., *Itinerary* (ed. Ch. Hughes). London, 1903.

MORYSON, F., *An Itinerary*. Glasgow, 1907.

MURATORI, L. A., *Del Governo della Peste*. Modena, 1714.

NICOLINI, F., *Peste e untori nei Promessi Sposi e nella realtà storica*. Bari, 1937.

NUTI, R., La popolazione di Prato, in *Archivio Storico Pratese*, 13 (1935).

OZANAM, J. A. F., *Histoire médicale générale et particulière des maladies épidemiques, contagieuses et épizootiques qui ont regné en Europe depuis les temps les plus reculés jusqu'à nos jours*. Paris, 1817.

PARENTI, G., *Prime ricerche sulla rivoluzione dei prezzi in Firenze*. Firenze, 1939.

PARISI, P., *Avvertimento sopra la peste*, Palermo, 1593.

POGGI, C., *Alcune notizie intorno la peste del 1630 in Como*. Como, 1886.

POLLITZER, R., *The Plague*. Geneve, 1954.

PONA, F., *Il gran contagio di Verona nel 1630*. Verona, 1727.

PRESOTTO, D., Genova 1656-1657. Cronache di una pestilenza, in *Atti Società Ligure di Storia Patria*, NS., 5 (1965).

PRINZING, F., *Epidemics resulting from wars*, ed. H. Westergaard. Oxford, 1916.

QUERINI, V., *Descrizione sulla peste che desolò Venezia nel 1630*. Venezia, 1831.

Ragguaglio dell'origine e giornalieri successi della gran peste seguita in Milano nell'anno 1629 al 1632. Milano, 1648.

RAVASINI, C., *Documenti sanitari, bolli e suggelli di disinfezione nel passato*. Trieste, 1958.

RIGHI, A., *Historia contagiosi morbi qui Florentiam depopulatus est anno 1630*. Firenze, 1633.

RIPAMONTI, J., *De Peste quae fuit anno 1630*. Milano, 1641.

RODENWALDT, L., *Pest in Venedig*. Heidelberg, 1952.

ROMANI, M. A., Aspetti dell' evoluzione demografica Parmense, in *Studi e ricerche della Facoltà di Economia e Commercio della Università di Parma*, vol. 7, Parma, 1970.

ROMANIN, S., *Storia documentata di Venezia*. Venezia, 1855.

RONDINELLI, F., *Relazione del Contagio stato in Firenze l'anno 1630 e 1633*. Firenze, 1634.

RUDEL, O., *Beiträge zur Geschichte der Medezin in Tirol*. Bolzano, 1925.

SCOTT, H. H., *A History of Tropical Medecine*. Baltimore, 1942.

SCOTTO, A., *Trattato istorico della peste dell'anno 1631*. Padova, 1633.

SELLA, D., La popolazione di Milano nei secoli XVI e XVII, in *Storia di Milano* ed. Treccani, vol. 12.

SERRA, G., *La Peste dell'anno 1630 nel Ducato di Modena*. Modena, 1960.

SEMBIANTI, P., Spigolature sulla peste e su altre malattie a Trento, in *Bollettino dell'Associazione Medica Tridentina*, 1924.

SETTALA, L., *De peste et pestiferis affectionibus*. Milano, 1622.

SHREWSBURY, J. F. D., *A History of Bubonic Plague in the British Isles*. Cambridge, 1970.

SIMPSON, W. J., *A Treatise on Plague*. Cambridge, 1905.

STICKER, G., *Abhandlungen aus der Seuchengeschichte und Seuchenlehre*, vol. I, *Die Pest*. Giessen, 1908.

SZTARONYI, V., *Ricordi storici di Riva al tempo della peste del 1630*. Riva del Garda, 1952.

TADINO, A., *Raguaglio dell'origine et giornali successi della gran peste*. Milano, 1648.

TARGIONI, L., Relazione della peste di Ferenze negli anni 1630 e 1631, in G. TARGIONI TOZZETTI, *Notizie degli aggrandimenti delle scienze fisiche in Toscana*, vol. 3.

TIRELLO, M., *La peste dell'Abbadia del Polesine . . . dell'anno 1630-1*. Rovigo, 1631.

TOLONE, M. DA, *Trattato politico da praticarsi in tempo di peste*. Genova, 1661.

VALENTE, A., La peste del 1576 in Milano, in *Archivio Storico Lombardo*, ser. 5, vol. 50 (1923).

WEBER, S., La peste del 1630 a Trento, in *Strenna Trentina*, January, 1926.

WU LIEN-TEH (ed.), *Manchurian Plague Prevention Service*. Memorial volume. Shanghai, 1934.

ZANELLI, A., Di alcune leggi suntuarie pistoiesi dal XIV al XVI secolo, in *Archivio Storico Italiano*, ser. 5, vol. 16 (1895).

INDEX

INDEX